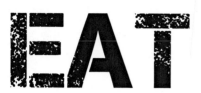

EAT FOR HEAT

THE METABOLIC APPROACH TO FOOD AND DRINK

Matt Stone

A proud presentation of:

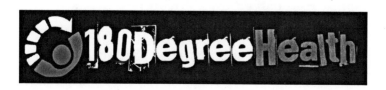

⸘ Published by Archangel Ink
ISBN 1484989317
ISBN-13: 978-148498319

DISCLAIMER

The material provided here is for educational and informational purposes only and is not intended as medical advice. The information contained in this book should not be used to diagnose or treat any illness, metabolic disorder, disease, or health problem. If you have developed a serious illness of some kind, the complexities of dealing with that disorder are best handled by your physician or other professional health care provider, whom you should also consult with before beginning any nutrition or exercise program. Use of the programs, advice, and other information contained in this book is at the sole choice and risk of the reader.

4

This book is not intended to increase and add on to the long list of health and dietary neuroticism that you may already possess. This book is not meant to be complex or confusing or to increasingly complicate the act of eating and drinking. It's meant to do the opposite actually – to simplify it. Make sure your implementation of any ideas gathered here is used in pursuit of simplicity.

Matt Stone; November 2012

Table of Contents

Introduction 7

E.C. – The Extra Cellular 13

Concentrate or Dilute 18

Warming Food, Cooling Food 34

Snacks 46

Circadian Rhythms 50

Adjusting Meal Schedule and Structure 55

The Overcompensation Effect 60

How Much Salt? 65

What to Drink? 74

6

Exercise 87

Disorders Most Likely to Be Affected..........................91

FAQ 96

Tools 104

References 106

About the Author...111

Introduction

E *at for Heat!* Provocative title isn't it? A tiny bit catchy perhaps? Yeah I know. I thought of it all by myself. Freaking genius.

Hmmm. Where to begin?

Well I guess I should be polite and introduce myself and give a little bit about where I'm coming from if this is the first book of mine that you've read. My name is Matt Stone. No, no initials or titles or formal certifications to go along with that. It's just me.

My interest in health dates back to childhood. As soon as I could read I was looking up and down the spines of my breakfast cereal to see what percentage of all my nutrients were found in the cereal. I wasn't into the bright colors or toys or any of that stuff. I wanted to eat healthfully, and chose my breakfast cereals based on how spectacular that spine looked. *Just Right* and *Total* were the obvious choices, with long lists of 100% on nearly every nutrient. That's what guided my choice of breakfast at least, long before I even sprouted pubes. I don't know where in the cosmos the health bug came from, but it's been with me as long as I can remember.

For whatever it's worth, I am a formally-educated writer, as in, I studied writing in college. As a writer you obviously have to pick a research focus. While I have several interests, human health has always been at or near the top. I decided to formally launch an "independent investigation" in 2006 and have since read over 300 books on the topic, perused hundreds of blogs, and read thousands of studies and research articles – all the while maintaining a blog of my own and communicating with thousands of other health nerds (40,000 comments and going) in pursuit of something valuable.

Most of the research I've done has funneled me closer and closer to one fundamental truth. That fundamental truth is that maintaining a high level of cellular energy production with a high metabolic rate and moderate levels of stress hormone exposure is the most useful and far-reaching health asset of them all. Every system of the body is influenced by the tug-of-war between energy and stress.

I won't go into all the details of why that is. I write about 1000 single-spaced pages per year and already have more than one book on the topic of cellular energy production – or metabolic rate if you are looking for a more familiar phrase.

Rather, this book is meant to build upon and expand the methodologies that I have devised for achieving this increase in metabolic rate over the years.

Eat for Heat represents, heading into 2013, what I think is one of the most useful, practical, and efficient ways of achieving a high metabolic rate. It's very simple.

And like most of what I write at 180DegreeHealth, much of the stuff you are about to read will challenge the status quo on certain pervasive health beliefs, such as "your pee should be clear," "drink 8, 8-ounce glasses water per day," "salt is bad for you," "fruits and vegetables are good for you," and more.

As a sneak preview, on the water front I will be challenging the idea that there should be some broad hydration prescription for the masses. General information is useless, and if it's taken too literally by a certain individual, it can be extraordinarily detrimental. Never before in history have humans been forcing themselves to drink so much water, or downing so many fluids in general. We drink to obtain sweetness, drugs, warmth when we're cold… lots of reasons other than thirst which is the ONLY biofeedback mechanism that should ever really be driving our drinking.

How much YOU should really drink on any given day at any given time will be the question that is answered to obscene thoroughness in this book. And we'll even go beyond that simple question to look at other factors to take into consideration. It's certainly not something you'll be able to look up on some chart on the internet somewhere, giving you the exact water requirement for your height, weight, and gender. No chart could ever achieve the precision that you'll be able to reach after reading this. No chart could even come close to the precision with which your own body is capable of managing this without the added guideposts we'll delve into.

In this book I don't plan on digging deep and exhaustively showing you all the research pointing to salt's benefits for example, or lack of need to suck down your body weight in water every day. I view such tactics as inefficient, and the results from that line of study to often be irrelevant to real-life, real-world health interventions with living, breathing, real people. Trying to make huge, sweeping intellectual arguments is tiring as well, and detracts from the simple basic insights that I've stumbled upon (which didn't happen as a result of perusing a bunch of studies or text books[1]).

What I'm saying is that I'm not going to waste a bunch of time talking about the history of how we came to fear salt as a society. I'm also not going to pinpoint study after study to coax you into feeling safe and secure about consuming salt liberally, or water sparingly. Maybe a couple, but not enough to blindside you into any one narrow line of thinking. It's simply not necessary, because with the implementation of some of these ideas I can virtually guarantee some of the quickest and most notable changes in your physiology that you've ever experienced. In all my years of study on the topic of human health, I can't say I've encountered anything quite as dramatic as the

---

[1] I did put a lab coat on and poked at some fetal pigs, but that was just to pass the time. I didn't learn anything from it. No I'm not serious. Yes I love using footnotes inappropriately. Are you still reading this?

things I've come to understand about regulating fluid concentrations in the body.

Fluid. That's what this book is all about. And it boils down to a concept so simple it's head-slapping. The food and fluids we take in can either increase or decrease the concentration of the fluids in our bodies. And this is more powerful and biologically significant than many of the miracle diets you've tried in the past, and more powerful than many of the miracle drugs and supplements you've popped. And it doesn't take long to kick in at all once you become aware of the concept and start applying it. The result? Higher core body temperature. Higher metabolic rate. Heat.

This is really the essence of what 180DegreeHealth is all about. This is simple, do-it-yourself health information that makes a tangible difference with an absolute minimum amount of effort. While I wouldn't expect miracles or set your expectations irrationally high, some of the things you will learn in this book should really help the systems of your body work better. And when the systems of the body work better, any number of different health problems and illnesses can improve.

Anyway, let's get on with it. I'm dying to tell everyone about this. While putting out a book on this topic might be a little premature, as my understanding of this is just beginning, I can't help but share what I've found so far – as soon as possible. I am one of the only people on earth with any conceptualization of this whatsoever, and one of the only people using dietary manipulation in this way. The sooner people hear about this and start catching onto it the better.

Before getting started, know that this is not some cure all. That's not the point, and it's important for everyone who reads health books and pursues different ideas to get beyond this naïve happily-ever-after fairy tale of perfect health and immortality. There's no such thing. Especially not in this day and age. This is merely a significant thing that you can tinker around with in addition to other basic health practices that you find realistic, sustainable, and enhancing to your life as a whole. Ultimately, an individual's health is either getting progressively better or progressively worse. Emphasize progress and dive into this with an open mind, as I have great confidence that this is one great, prior-to-now undiscovered secret to getting back in the improving health category without making any other dramatic changes.

E.C. – The Extra Cellular

Remember when E.T. was laying by the creek after a hard night. Little wrinkly bastard looked pretty rough. All pale and what not. Guarantee you his extracellular fluid was really diluted. His blood volume? Down. I don't know why they didn't put him on an I.V. when they captured him, pumping him full of saline until he got a nice rosy color back into his tissues. That is, after all, what happens when you build back the extracellular fluid, including the volume of the blood.

Extracellular fluid, also known as interstitial fluid, is the fluid in your body that is NOT inside any cells. It's the fluid outside of cells, and runs, in a typical person, somewhere around 15 liters and includes the blood.

As we age, extracellular fluid decreases and blood volume decreases on a pound for pound basis. In other words, kids have the most in proportion to their body weight. The elderly have the least. And the concentration of that fluid seems to be on a downward trajectory as well, becoming ever-more diluted. This seems to accompany the declining metabolic rate with aging, as hypothyroidism and diluted body fluids are apparently related.

A falling blood volume is a hallmark of aging. Blood volume is really important. One of the most powerful medical interventions ever discovered was pumping really salty water into the bloodstream of sick people to increase blood volume, vascularity, and normalize blood pressure. They even created a motto which we'll delve into the significance of later in terms of when to stop expanding blood volume... "Open up, and fill up. Stop when the feet get warm." http://www.ncbi.nlm.nih.gov/pmc/articles/PMC1701158/pdf/brmedj02298-0064a.pdf

Not to go off on a tangent here, but try pumping pure water into someone's veins. You'll frickin' kill 'em I bet. Yet, we are instructed to drink a couple quarts of pure water daily and restrict salt to the bare minimum. Great. Thanks mainstream. Okay I'll back off the tangent and save more of that ranting for later...

None of this is exactly rocket science. Common sense will tell you that the elderly steadily see a decrease in proper blood circulation, and much of this has to do with a falling blood volume. With age, hands and feet and other peripheral areas (such as the epidermis) get colder and drier. That's why old people gravitate towards places like Arizona and Florida, where I live. A guy in my building died this week for crying out loud. Another old lady fell and broke her arm. Old I tell ya. They love this Florida place. I don't know how I ended up here. Oh yeah, I remember. To be close to my sick, old grandfather that lives here.

As a general rule, anything that typically falls with age you want to keep from falling. Anything that rises with age, like triglycerides or blood pressure, you want to keep from rising. All of that is statistical and lacks individuality, but in general principle you want to avoid the things that happen with aging because aging, quite frankly, represents a descent in functionality. Falling blood volume, a decrease in total body water content, a decrease in the salinity of the extracellular fluid – those are the things that we're looking to target with some of the simple tweaks discussed in this book.

Aside from all that, I think what the basic principle I've stumbled upon when it comes to making a few changes in diet and drink, is how to increase the concentration of the body fluids. By an increase in concentration, I mean more minerals like calcium and sodium found in the extracellular fluid in proportion to water, and perhaps sugar as well, although it's hard to say exactly how sugar factors in biochemically. But it does play a vital role, as the desired objective is virtually impossible on a low-carb diet in my experience.

This may seem like a far out concept, but picture your body filled with nutritious, high-octane, electrically conductive fluids. Things work better, and your cells have the ability to produce more energy at the cellular level. Once again, I don't have a perfect scientific understanding of what's going on inside of the body or the cells with some of the tactics we'll be discussing.

Rather, this is all an attempt at providing a rational explanation for what I have found to be true and very helpful for increasing body heat, body temperature, and the physiological functions related to them – which includes just about everything, as every system of the body is dependent on the quality of energy produced by the mitochondria.

It is my belief that the things discussed here must somehow perform this feat because of the reliability that changes such as an increase in the warmth of the hands and feet and body temperature in general occur. Accompanying this are typical pro-metabolism changes such as increased skin moisture, rapid growth of hair and nails, increased sweating, a calmer mood, and many others.

And because these changes are stimulated primarily by changing the concentration of certain foodstuffs, salt in particular, in relation to total fluid intake, it stands to reason that this is helping to expand blood volume and increase the concentration of the extracellular fluid. That's the only reasonable explanation I've been able to come up with thus far.

The concentration of the urine is one of the best outwardly indicators that we have access to, and because of my studies of nutrition's impact on the concentration of the urine, I have come to think that the concentration of the urine is a pretty good indicator of the concentration of the primary body fluids as well. There is at least a correlation. That much I'm sure about.

But like I said, this is not a big book of scientific speculation. No one, including myself, needs a complex understanding of biochemistry in order to implement a few changes and see the results. It was, I thought, at least worth mentioning that it probably is the concentration of the extracellular fluid that we are manipulating here, and that this is quite physiologically significant. It was also worth it to mention *E.T.*, because *E.T.* was an 80's movie – 1982 to be exact. And it will be a cold day in hell when I write a book without randomly referencing an 80's film, music group, television show, fashion trend, toy, or otherwise.

Concentrate or Dilute

So, now that we've gotten that brief introduction into extracellular fluid out of the way, let's get down to the business of specifics. The most important element that I want people to understand is that the body can be "overhydrated" in a sense. That's really not the best descriptive word. A better word to describe it is "diluted." You guys hopefully know what it means to dilute right? Well if not, that's what Google is for.

I put an emphasis on the overly-diluted side of things for several reasons…

There is more societal paranoia about dehydration, and there's next to nothing about the dangers of overconsumption of fluids. Yes, we know dehydration is bad. It will give you a headache, ruin your athletic performance progressively as it becomes more severe, make you more likely to overheat on a hot day, and could kill you… yes, kill you… so please don't take anything to extremes here – the point is to achieve

optimal balance and take advantage of that inner
stability. The body loves that balance and stability
stuff. But yes, I feel compelled to show the other side
of the story. Hey, it's 180DegreeHealth. It's what I do.

My research has progressively led me towards the
central importance of metabolic rate in health, the
dangers of dieting, and so on. And those with a low
metabolism typically have weakened body fluids with a
greater tendency to become dangerously diluted –
enough to trigger immediately tangible symptoms.
Plus, I attract a lot of people with low metabolic rates,
so I feel it's a good fit for my typical audience member.

Overhydration is MUCH more common in the
water-loving, dehydration-panicked, salt-phobic realm
of the modern internet-scouring health nerd, and the
symptoms of overhydration/dilution trump that of
being mildly dehydrated by a long shot – typically
existing on a near constant basis and creating suffering
daily at one or more points during the day.

You are less likely to become dehydrated in my
estimation, mostly because the thirst mechanism is a lot
stronger than the "not thirst" mechanism. If you
become dehydrated you'll get too thirsty to ignore it.
It's easier to ignore the signal that says "Nah, I'm not
that thirsty right now" and keep on chugging away,
especially when many fluids these days serve some
other purpose – like satisfying a sweet craving,
providing a hit of aspartame or caffeine, or warming
you up on a cold day.

But ultimately you will need to determine for
yourself whether you are more likely to need to

concentrate the fluids in your body or dilute the fluids in your body on any given day, at any given time, or just in a general sense. Before going into detail about how to determine such a thing, now seems as good a time as any to mention rule #1, a rule far more important than anything else we'll discuss in the rest of this chapter – and maybe the whole book actually…

Do NOT drink when you are NOT thirsty.

Especially fluids that lack salt and sugar like tea, coffee, diet drinks, and plain water. The only time this can be beneficial is when you are about to exercise or go out and do strenuous work at very high temperatures. In other words, drinking when not thirsty is only potentially beneficial in anticipation of losing a bunch of water. Forcing yourself to meet some quota of fluids, drinking because you think you should, having a hot beverage because you are cold – this is very powerfully depleting and can trigger some real health problems in someone in a compromised metabolic condition.

If everyone obeyed this one simple rule there would hardly be a need to write this book. But, bless us, we're humans after all. We have these big brains that can do some neat things, but leave it to us to do something as stupid as drink when we're not thirsty. No other creature does this. No other creature is so removed from its own instinctual programming to the point of accidentally overdrinking. The mechanisms of the body generally prevent such a thing. Intellectual interference between our bodies' needs and what we think are our bodies' needs forms a barrier that can be quite problematic, especially when it comes to flooding out the electrical supply of our entire inner metropolis.

Now that this one major point is behind us, let's move on…

By my best estimation, the most practical indicator of whether we need to concentrate our body fluids or dilute them is to examine the one body fluid we examine multiple times each day – our urine.
The big question is, how concentrated should our urine be? One indicator of urine concentration is a measurement known as specific gravity. That would be a number that increases as the amount of dissolved particles in the urine increases. Normal appears to be between a specific gravity range of 1.012 to 1.030. A practical way to measure this, and a tool that I used extensively to arrive at some of these conclusions, is to use an instrument known as a refractometer. The unit of measurement with a refractometer is called "brix." A specific gravity of 1.012 to 1.030 translates to roughly 3 to 7.5 brix.

When I first encountered the use of the refractometer I was really blown away. Feelings of cold hands and feet, bad moods, and other very mild symptoms occurred consistently when my urine brix had fallen below 2.0 or was rapidly descending. By descending I mean that I could take a urine sample when I felt a lull in mood and energy levels coming on in the normal 4-5 range, but an hour later would have a sudden urge to urinate and it would be somewhere between 1-2. I tested to the point where I could actually predict when my urine concentration was about to get weak just based upon my biofeedback. I even got to where I could guess within a point of what my urine concentration was going to be just based on how I felt. It was a remarkable revelation.

Even more remarkable was seeing how severe the symptoms of others were who had worse metabolic problems than I. Symptoms of nausea, vomiting, seizure, headache, migraine, insomnia, rapid or erratic pulse, anxiety attacks, and so forth typically coincided with bouts of frequent urination with a brix below 1, or sometimes as low as a completely flat 0. Likewise I noticed that stress such as arguments, excessive exercise, sleep loss, or fasting triggered lower-density urine. All my observations were enough to arrive at a great level of confidence that urine concentration was significant, and normalizing it could indeed eliminate many health problems almost overnight.

This actually isn't some big secret. It is scientifically known and understood that having overly-diluted body fluids can lead to basically every symptom I just listed. The condition (of diluted fluids) is referred to as "water intoxication" and also referred to as "hyponatremia," or low salt levels in the blood. From the Wikipedia page on water intoxication…

"At the onset of this condition, fluid outside the cells has an excessively low amount of solutes (such as sodium (hyponatremia) and other electrolytes) in comparison to that inside the cells causing the fluid to shift through (via osmosis) into the cells to

balance its concentration. This causes the cells to swell. In the brain, this swelling increases intracranial pressure (ICP). It is this increase in pressure which leads to the first observable symptoms of water intoxication: headache, personality changes, changes in behavior, confusion, irritability, and drowsiness. These are sometimes followed by difficulty breathing during exertion, muscle weakness, twitching, or cramping, nausea, vomiting, thirst, and a dulled ability to perceive and interpret sensory information. As the condition persists papillary and vital signs may result including bradycardia and widened pulse pressure. The cells in the brain may swell to the point where blood flow is interrupted resulting in cerebral edema. Swollen brain cells may also apply pressure to the brain stem causing central nervous system dysfunction. Both cerebral edema and interference with the central nervous system are dangerous and could result in seizures, brain damage, coma or death."

Bradycardia by the way presents symptoms such as "fatigue, weakness, dizziness, lightheadedness, fainting, chest discomfort, palpitations, or shortness of breath." Hyponatremia is described with identical symptoms to water intoxication, and has been linked to things such as increased bone fracture in the elderly, just to name one of the many negative things I'm sure they will discover in the coming decades…
http://www.springerlink.com/content/g1x5416r835816 32/?MUD=MP

Knowing that there are millions of people out there who deal with many of these symptoms and many others that aren't recognized or listed above on a daily basis, this was an absolute gold mine of a discovery. The solution is simple for most, and many cases of people who are chronically experiencing all of the above symptoms will respond fantastically. This is alone worth getting a book into print.

But I also noticed the metabolism connection to urine concentration. Metabolism has been an interest of mine since early on in my health exploration, and gradually became the epicenter of my research focus after developing a reliable method to increase it. Three of the best outwardly indicators of the health of one's metabolic rate, although they all have their drawbacks, are body temperature, general feeling of body warmth, and the warmth of the hands and feet. The warmth of the hands and feet is of particular interest because it signifies a calm nervous system with generally less stress hormone exposure – as an activation of the stress side of the nervous system causes blood vessels in the periphery (hands, feet, ears, tip of nose) to close. Reducing stress hormone exposure appears, by most accounts, to be a good thing with far-reaching health benefits. Spending more time with hands and feet warm, as opposed to cold, therefore represents a very significant physiological change taking place underneath the surface.

Body warmth is generally much higher when urine concentration is higher. Likewise, those with very low density urine often have a tendency to feel extremely cold, especially in the hands and feet. This made me think back to some past extreme dieting errors that left me squirting clear-as-water piss every 20 minutes – just from having some oatmeal cooked in water, not even actually drinking water straight. Eating a high fruit diet reliably had this impact as well, and proponents of a fruit-based diet actually recommend peeing clear and even go so far as to suggest that a person is not healthy unless they are getting up and urinating at least a few times every night (WTF?).

Anyway, a guide to not only overcoming many of the symptoms that we've discussed already, but also investing in spending time in a metabolically enhanced, low stress state, is the concentration of the urine. No of course this is not the pee all end all to health. But there is power in regulating the basic systems of the body. Normalizing any system, like the concentration of the fluids in your body, normalizes many systems. When systems are balanced and there is stability within, you function better and have less chance of getting sick in the short and long term.

While I wouldn't discourage anyone from using a refractometer as I did to better learn how your body functions, it certainly isn't necessary to use any fancy equipment or play with your whiz, despite its inherent fun-ness. Yellow is good. Clear is bad. Very pale or light yellow can be on the cusp of trouble. Very dark yellowish orange, or having urine so strong and concentrated it actually burns your piss pipe (the uh, urethra I think they call it… do you concur doctor?), is probably overdoing it a bit.

I do prefer the biofeedback I experience by keeping urine concentration more on the high side though, I must say. I sweat more, sleep better, feel calm, have faster growing hair and nails, my skin moisture is much higher – all positive metabolic signs.

While there is limited study into more concentrated urine and its possible benefits, one thing that I did find reassuring were some studies brought up not too long ago by several prominent alternative health icons, such as Dr. Mercola and the Weston A. Price Foundation, on the subject of salt.

For example, low sodium levels in the urine (sodium content in urine closely parallels the brix value or overall concentration) have an association with higher rates of myocardial infarction, although there's no telling how relevant this particular study is to the average Joe...
http://www.ncbi.nlm.nih.gov/pubmed?term=%22Hyper tension%22%5BJour%5D+AND+1995%5Bpdat%5D+ AND+urinary+sodium&TransSchema=title&cmd=detai lssearch

A far more shocking and promising study was published in 2011...
http://jama.jamanetwork.com/article.aspx?articleid=899 663

In this study, several thousand Europeans were followed for eight years, and they kept track of total mortality and morbidity (death and illness) rates for everyone involved – breaking them into 3 categories based on sodium excretion in the urine. In the third with the highest sodium excretion in the urine (and therefore highest urine concentration), 10 died. But there were 50 deaths in the clear-pissing group. 5 times as many deaths! There were 24 deaths in the moderate urine sodium group. The higher the urine sodium excretion, the lower the death rate. Those aren't mild,

accidental, or by-chance numbers differences either.
Those are huge differences and very statistically
significant. You hardly ever hear about something
quite so statistically different just based on something
like urine sodium excretion.

Anyway, a few studies shouldn't make us all lose our
minds with thoughts of immortality. But I bring them
up for reassurance. In the articles that I saw the last
study mentioned, they were used in defense of
consuming plenty of salt. And sure, your urine will
have more sodium in it if you consume more salt,
generally-speaking. But of course the concentration of
the urine or its sodium content isn't dependent solely
on salt intake, but also on total fluid intake and other
factors like metabolic rate and carbohydrate
consumption. It's important that the net result of all
your food and fluids is the equivalent of what's called a
"hypertonic solution," or solution with a greater
concentration than normal body fluids if you are
looking for metabolism increase. And research into the
powerful benefit of hypertonic solutions in the right
context are even more reassuring, such as the use of
hypertonic solutions to decrease inflammation for
example…
http://scienceblog.com/56744/

So I guess without further ado let's talk in plain and
simple terms about when you need to concentrate your
body fluids, including your urine…
In terms of getting a general sense, you should urinate
about once every four hours during the day I would
say, and none during your sleep at night. The ideal

range might be 4-6 eliminations in each 24 hour cycle. But like I mentioned earlier, you want these as evenly-spaced as possible, with a consistent color and concentration, for reassurance that your inner environment is stable. Stability is extremely powerful. So that is the general goal.

Some other indicators that your urine concentration might be too weak on a chronic basis, is having cold hands and feet all the time, a low body temperature, low or inconsistent energy levels or chronic fatigue, a tendency towards anxiety or panic attacks, migraines or seizures, bouts of blurred vision or brain fog, insomnia, mood swings including irritability, headaches, dry skin, poorly-growing hair and nails, dry mouth or excessive thirst, erratic heartbeat, abnormal blood pressure, constipation or Irritable Bowel Syndrome, and many others yet to be revealed.

Interestingly, I think many of the problems that people assume to be "hypoglycemia" are actually hyponatremia, or perhaps even something less detectable than varying blood concentrations of any given substance (as in, weakened/diluted extracellular fluid). I found it interesting that early works on hypoglycemia, such as Abrahamson and Pezet's *Body, Mind, and Sugar* (1951) identified alcohol, soft drinks, and coffee as primary triggers of hypoglycemia, all of which are often consumed in excess of physiological fluid needs and spark frequent urination and accompanying symptoms (again, the severity of the symptoms depends in large part on how metabolically strong the person urinating frequently is).

So those are some of the indicators that you may need to increase the concentration of your fluids. But that's really just in terms of doing that in a general sense. As we'll spend more than ample time discussing later, keeping your body fluids in the ideal "zone" is not something that you really do in a general way, but in a precise way with vigilance throughout each and every day. Most people don't have overly concentrated or overly diluted body fluids all the time. Most people seesaw back and forth between overly concentrated and overly diluted, and that brings us to what you could consider to be rule #2...

Any time you pee clear, have a particularly strong urge to urinate that strikes you suddenly, urinate several times in rapid succession, or pee an abnormally large amount – eat a salty carbohydrate-rich snack or meal as soon as possible.

Because we have radically varying hormonal rhythms and radical variance in our diets and lifestyles, you may only have a tendency to have cold hands and feet, symptoms of diluted fluids, and clear, sudden, or frequent urination at certain times of the day, but not all the time. That's typical.

Let's say for example you normally go to bed at 11pm. But you stayed up to 2am one night, hopefully because of your rock star sexual capabilities and not because there was a *Lizard Lick Towing* marathon goin' down on TruTv. You get 5 hours of sleep that night instead of 8+. You'll notice that your tendency to crash out and urinate more frequently, with a lower body temperature and colder hands and feet, is much greater on less sleep. You have to adjust your eating and drinking that day to accommodate this stress.

Another scenario I see frequently is people having absolutely no problems all day long, and then, at about 9pm commences a very powerful physical decline. Body temperature plummets, hands and feet get freezing cold, and the frequent urination commences. Yeah I'm talking to you Ms. Two pairs of socks to sleep in every night. You lie in bed but forget it. You keep having to get up every 20 minutes to pee. And you have to pee REALLY BAD, but hardly anything comes out and it's as clear as water. You thought you were the only one. There are actually lots of people out there with this problem, and adjusting the timing, type, and quantity of food and fluid intake during the day can eliminate this problem – as well as the problems that it causes, like sleep loss, or just crappy sleep in general with a lot of wakeups, nightmares, and general brain overactivity (including night terrors and talking and twitching and all that stuff that annoys your partner and decreases his or her sleep quality as well).

Anyway, those are just two scenarios. There are many more that I hope to address with specificity. The point is that you have to keep an awareness of this in the back of your mind, and make tiny adjustments in accordance with your own personal rhythms that keep you in a stable and balanced state as much as possible. Avoid all crashes, or respond to them quickly with carbs and salt, and do so consistently and the cumulative effect will most likely yield a lot of health improvements. At least it has in my experience with it thus far.

When do you need to actually dilute your fluids? This has come up a lot, as the strategies I lay out later are so powerful it doesn't take long to actually get to the point where you are overdoing it. Uncomfortably hot hands and feet are a sign that you need to drink some fluids, and ease up on the salt and heaviness of your meals at the time of day you tend to experience this – for most this surfaces at night (and sometimes causes restless legs). Other signs are an extremely heavy, uncomfortable pulse – this I believe is from your blood volume actually expanding too much, which causes the left ventricle of your heart to have to work way too hard. Headache accompanying the warmth in the hands and feet is also usually from overly concentrated body fluids.

And the weirdest "side effect" of having overly concentrated body fluids that I've encountered is what I describe as the "doubling of gravity" effect. Go really overboard on salt consumption for example, and you may be one of the unlucky ones to experience this. It's really bizarre, and "doubling of gravity" is the best way to describe it. It's like an immovable tiredness but without feeling drowsy. It really feels like you are wearing a knight's armor or something. And if you aren't wearing armor, about all the strength you can muster is shouting a few insults at your enemy, standing up slowly, pointing your sword at him, and saying "Drop. Your. Sword" before collapsing. I know I sound psycho elaborating upon this in such great detail, and referencing an 80's movie yet again, but if anyone feels it I want them to recognize what's going on and not keep on dumping in the salt to try to make it go away.

Keep in mind that extreme dieters and those with a history of eating disorders are the ones most likely to experience a lot of what this book addresses, and well, in my experience those with such personality traits have a tendency to eat their body weight in salt and fear drinking more than a thimble-sized glass of water at first until they get this dialed in.

Anyway, those are a few guideposts to familiarize yourself with on when to dilute and when to concentrate. This chapter is droning on and on and getting unorganized, so I'm going to end it and subdivide the application of this stuff into a new chapter or two.

But before moving on let's shave this all down into the most simple concept we can. The simple version of all this crap I've been saying is this... We'll call this Rule #3 I guess?

When you are cold, especially in the hands and feet, your urine is clear, the urge to urinate is strong, or you are peeing frequently... YOU NEED TO EAT MORE AND DRINK LESS When you are hot, especially in the hands and feet, your urine is dark or you haven't peed in a really

**long time… YOU NEED TO EAT LESS AND
DRINK MORE**

I told you man. Groundbreaking, earth-shattering stuff
here right. Oh yeah, I thought of this all by myself.
Self-taught. Not one lesson Pops!

Warming Food, Cooling Food

To help people who I have communicated with in person to better grasp this concept, I've come up with a few simple examples. When it comes to a meal or snack that you consume having a net cooling or net warming effect, it's not just about how much salt or how many calories or how much water you drink with the meal. All that matters, as I touched on earlier, is that the total sum of the food and fluids that you consume yield the equivalent of either a hypertonic, isotonic, or hypotonic solution.

As a quick primer, saline that they give in intravenous therapy is called "isotonic" when it contains 9 grams of salt per liter. This is a rough, a very rough, approximation of what the normal concentration of the extracellular fluid is. A hypertonic solution would have more than 9 grams per liter, or be a stronger, more concentrated solution. A hypotonic solution would have less than 9 grams per liter, and be a weaker, more diluted solution. I suppose this will serve as a reasonable baseline. We are not going to calculate anything. Don't worry. This is just to provide a stronger conceptual grasp of what the hell it is I'm saying here.

So one thing I often say is…

"You can eat a whole entire pizza, but if you drink a gallon of water with it you're likely to be freezing cold and peeing your brains out an hour later. Eat a single slice of pizza but only have a couple sips of a beverage with it and you'll be warm and toasty later."

You can see the basic concept at play here, and you can experiment with this a little bit yourself to validate it if you want. The guiding idea is manipulating the ratio of food to fluids. I think when you start tinkle tinkering it will become obvious.

Likewise, I also often mention something like…

"If you wake up and eat a bowl of watery oatmeal for breakfast with a glass of milk and 3 big slices of watermelon you'll be peeing and freezing all morning."

This is, of course, because the water content is so high – especially in proportion to the amount of salt in a breakfast like that.

Or…

"It doesn't matter how much watermelon you eat, it will never make you warm. The amount of calories and sodium in proportion to the water content makes it impossible."

So anyway, what I'm getting at is that some foods are warming. Some are cooling. Drinks of all kinds are generally cooling unless it is extremely calorie dense, like half and half with molasses added ("halfasses" I call it – yes it's better than it sounds, and yes I am hilarious thank you for noticing).

The beauty of this revelation, I think, is being able to achieve the net-warming effect of eating – something that is not an easy task for someone with a suppressed metabolic rate, and keep the stress system suppressed and the metabolism high. Well, not only that you can achieve that, but that you can do it without necessarily blatantly overconsuming food to the point of being stuffed – a tactic that I relied on exclusively before coming across this increasingly precise way to do business (you should still eat to fullness though, no matter what).

The most warming substances, in my experience, are sugar, starch, and salt – with saturated fat as an honorable mention. Well, any fat is warming because of the calorie-density of fat, but dairy, red meat, cocoa, and coconut fats (the most saturated sources) theoretically should have the best long-term preservation of metabolism and mitochondrial energy production. Thus was born the...

"Anti-Stress S's" – Sugar, Starch, Salt, and Saturated fat.

And that's just in terms of food. Other anti-stress S's include sleep, sun, saltwater (as in hanging out on the beach, but may also include salt-water baths and the actual salty water itself), and perhaps sex (although that depends on the context).

None of these really work in isolation, not even the salt – as we need carbohydrates to actually assimilate the salt, which is why rehydration drinks contain both salts/electrolytes and glucose. I find they work best when combined together. They taste better combined together too – all the edible S's that is, which fosters greater calorie consumption and subsequently obtaining the necessary amount of calories required to obtain or maintain a healthy metabolism.
Not everyone has universally noticed the warming effects of any one type of food as was revealed in a survey-esque article I wrote entitled "What Gets You Hot?" But generally the yummy foods, and yummy meals get it done the best. You'll note that meals that include a combination of several of the items below have the greatest warming effect.

Some of the superstars are:

Cheese – with the high calorie density, high salt content, and extremely low water content it's hard to go wrong with cheese, or things that have lots of cheese on them like pizza, grilled cheese sandwiches, or cheeseburgers

Coconut – Coconut oil is renowned for its ability to assist with metabolic rate and body heat, but any source of coconut will do. The medium-chain saturated fatty acids seem to be the active warming ingredient. Coconut is of course very calorie dense with a low water content, and cooking foods in oil of any kind increases the calorie to water ratio

Chocolate – Calorie dense with a low water content and some sugar in it too. I can't overdo it on the chocolate or my bed sheets get drenched with sweat

Flours – Flours made from grains, wheat of course being the most common, have very high calorie density and no water content at all until some liquid is added in the preparation of things like bread, crackers, pastries, tortillas, cookies, and so on. With the high starch levels and calorie density, and their palatability, flour-products are generally very warming

Red Meat – It's not always warming, but generally the fattier cuts of red meat like beef and lamb are very warming. Fatty red meat is very calorie dense, and it also absorbs a phenomenal amount of salt before it becomes disgustingly salty. A double cheeseburger at Mickey D's has more salt than an entire large bag of Sea Salt Kettle Chips, yet the chips actually taste saltier

Potatoes – Potatoes are not as calorie dense as other foods, but with their high starch levels and the large quantity of salt they require to be maximally palatable, potatoes fried in coconut oil or mashed with butter are an old warming standby in my house. All varieties of sweet potatoes and yams are great too, as are the less commonly used tubers like yucca and taro

Soy sauce – Soy sauce is very warming due to its extreme saltiness, and the taste is outstanding, which fosters a total salt consumption that is much higher than when you use regular table salt to season your food

Ice cream – Ice cream packs quite a lot of energy per unit of volume, and lots of sugar without the high water content of fruit or juice. It's cold, but most feel very warm after eating some ice cream and similar desserts like cheesecake, panna cotta, or pudding

Other desserts – Any of the typical dessert-type foods, including cookies, pastries, pies, cakes, and just about anything you can think of are extremely warming due to the palatability, low water content, and high sugar content of most desserts

Now on to the cooling foods/substances…

Water – Of course. The only time water seems to have a warming effect is when you are truly dehydrated and your stress system is activated by it. Otherwise it is generally cooling

Coffee and tea – I don't think these are exceptionally cooling, but tend to have a cooling effect because people consume them when they are cold and are hoping to warm up. In the short-term the temperature of them is warming, but it perpetuates the coldness. The lower the metabolic rate, the higher the desire to drink warm fluids and to take in stimulants, so one should really use caution when it comes to consuming coffee and tea regularly

Soft Drinks – Soft drinks are generally considered to be the single most fattening substance in the modern diet. That's a bold proclamation, as no food or drink in isolation is truly inherently fattening. But soft drinks do encourage drinking beyond thirst, drinking beyond thirst does lower body temperature (which reduces metabolic rate and calorie burn at rest by a substantial amount), and anything that lowers calorie burn while providing a lot of calories to go with it is a prime suspect in the separation in equality between calories burned and calories consumed that leads to changes in body weight

Juice – Juice shares many similarities to soft drinks and in my experience is even more cooling than soft drinks, perhaps due to the high potassium content of most juices

Diet Drinks – Diet drinks are the granddaddy of them all. Sweeteners like aspartame are extremely sweet and also cause excitation in the brain. Throw in some caffeine and you've got something very attractive. I notice that it's very common for diet drink consumers to consume outrageous quantities, and diet drink consumption has been tied to many symptoms indistinguishable from the symptoms of excess water consumption – like headaches, migraines, and seizures. Diet drinks are worse because they provide no sugar, unlike juice and sugared soft drinks. The cooling effect is similar to water, but the qualities of diet drinks foster much greater consumption beyond physiological need

Lowfat Milk – Eat a few bowls of cereal (who eats just one?) with whole milk – you might be warm. Eat a few bowls of cereal with skim milk and forget about it. The removal of saturated fats and most of the calories seems to make skim milk function less like a meal, and more like a glass of water consumed beyond physiological fluid needs

Soup – Soup is warming short-term because of the temperature. But soup can be cooling too. It's very filling. To actually get enough calories from most soups you would have to consume far too much fluid.

But soups like the potato soup I make, cooked in whole milk, with lots of added salt, butter, and cheese is actually warming. But those things have to be added to keep it from being cooling. The same could be said for oatmeal and other porridges

Fruit – Fruit, with its high water content, low calorie-density, and high potassium to sodium ratio is amongst the most cooling of all foods. A little is fine. Going beyond physiological fluid needs with fruit is extremely cooling. Same could be said of smoothies, especially ones made with just frozen fruit and juice, or lowfat yoghurt or soy milk or something. Brrrr. Would be nice in the tropics and in the summer when it's actually advantageous to be cooler though. Adding salt to fruit, as is done where I grew up with things like citrus and watermelon, helps a lot. But that can be said of any of the things listed on this page

Vegetables – Like fruit, vegetables can be very cooling for the same reasons. Few people overconsume vegetables, but it can be done, especially if you are doing a lot of juicing

These are decent lists to start with, but even so, looking at these lists doesn't really tell the whole story of what I'm trying to convey. Not at all really, because no one just sits down and eats nothing but fruit. Well, some do. But anyone remotely in tune with their body's needs, cravings, and biofeedback will have gotten past such a phase hopefully.

This list is in no way an attempt to steer you towards the warming list at the exclusion of the cooling list. If you do that you'll croak. You can't just eat pizza and cookies and chug a glass of soy sauce and not take any complementary fluids with it. The higher your metabolic rate, and if you do any strenuous exercise (which you probably should once your health is fairly stable), the more fluids and thus cooling foods you will need to consume.

Now don't freak out on me because all the foods on the warming list are "bad" for you. Such foods can be taken to excess no doubt, but such foods are incredibly therapeutic for the journey from having a low metabolism to a normal or above-normal metabolic rate. The irony is that if you are in rough metabolic shape – let's say you have dieted extensively, you will actually need to eat "unhealthy" food for a while in order to graduate to eating a "healthy diet." I know that sounds weird, but try dieting. Does it increase or decrease your cravings for the items on list 1 or list 2? I rest my case. And this is actually a beautiful thing that your body does to save you from yourself. Binging on junk food is actually what your body does to heal itself from the harms various forms of self-deprecating eating and exercise programs deliver.

I can still hear you going off on a tangent about the stuff you've read about fructose, the processing of table salt, the glutamic acid in soy sauce, the hormones in ice cream, the evil villainous gluten, the lack of vitamins or fiber in white flour, or otherwise. As someone who spent the better part of a decade wrapped up in such relative minutiae, I highly encourage you to let go of a lot of that fluff and give this a try. Your fears and the things you are ideologically tethered to from excess internet health reading will hopefully fade pretty quickly until you are eating a more sustainable and socially-reasonable diet, and feeling a heck of a lot better than you were when intellectualizing every last detail of your food choices.

If you're not hip to that, that's fine too. As Uncle Rico said in *Napolean Dynamite*, "Stop wishing, and call me when you're ready[2]."

But regardless of what you believe, and what you feel is appropriate and "safe" for you to eat personally, you can still of course apply the basic principles we're discussing here. You can eat all the grassfed yak butter and goji juice and Himalayan beetle pus and tree bark that you want. Just put some soy sauce on it and stop drinking so much f'ing water.

What I meant by putting together these lists are to help you become aware of the connections, and learn to balance things appropriately. Here are some examples of how you might actually think about things as you go to construct a meal...

If you are going to eat oatmeal for example, that's absolutely fine. But if you eat it plain, cooked in water with no salt added, it will tank your metabolism. Try cooking it in milk and adding sugar, salt, and butter. Problem solved. Net effect: warming.

Likewise, if you are going to eat oatmeal for breakfast, don't make it too watery like soup. Also take note of the fact that there is a lot of fluid in the

---

[2] This was used in the movie in reference to natural breast enhancement, which is fitting because eating lots of the foods in list #1 will certainly increase your breast size. My girlfriend's up a couple cup sizes.

oatmeal. Oatmeal is a water-rich food. You wouldn't want to complement the meal with other water-rich things like a big glass of milk and 2 oranges, or a smoothie let's say. You might be better off complementing it with something very salty with a low water content, like a couple slices of cheese and only a small handful of fruit – added to the oatmeal perhaps. That would be a great warming meal, and be complete with sufficient calories and the full constellation of S foods – sugar, starch, salt, and saturated fat. This same line of thinking can be applied to all kinds of porridges, breakfast cereal with milk (don't drown it!), soups, etc.

Or let's say that you really feel that fruit is a healthy food for you, and you like it. Well, that may or may not be true depending on who you are and what kind of metabolic state you're in. The main thing is that you don't wash your metabolism out and activate your stress system. You could sprinkle some salt on it, or let it marinate in a pinch of salt. Trust me, some strawberries or peaches marinated in a little salt won't hurt the flavor.

Or you could do the same with sugar – put a little sugar or maple syrup over the fruit and let it marinate for a little bit.

Or you could have a fingerlickin' grilled cheese sandwich laced with salted butter along with your fruit, adding salt, starch, fat, and calories to your fruit to make a complete meal.

Better yet, do all those things.

What really matters is that you don't overdo the fluids, or at least that you become cognizant of how food interacts with your body to the extent that you can start mastering it and staying in a nice high metabolism, low stress "zone" all the time.

The biggest help is just making sure to salt food until it tastes "just right." Eat until you are full and satisfied of a variety of foods to ensure adequate calorie intake. Then drink or eat something juicy like fruit when you are thirsty but never beyond your physical thirst unless it's in anticipation of a hot day outdoors or a tough workout or something. That's really about all there is to it. I know it sounds simple but that's the point. The answers to better health, I have found, are mostly found in the simple realm. And there is no better guide to anything than our own tastes, appetites, and thirsts. Disobeying our body's cries for certain things, overriding our instincts, and exerting stubborn willpower is where we create the most damage, generally-speaking.

Okay, you should be getting it now. Don't forget you can overdo the warming stuff too, especially when you are already in a warm and toasty state. There are some more interesting tidbits to add, and more discussion before we can even think of wrapping this thing up though. More to come…

Snacks

If you could summarize the overall goal of this stuff, I would say it is to keep the inner environment of the body in a stable, consistent state. The body just works better in that state, and that seems to be its general agenda. In achieving that, I find snacks to be instrumental, especially for those in a compromised metabolic state who often feel like they are on a biochemical rollercoaster.

The most important use of the snack is to lift your body out of an active stress event. It takes a surprisingly miniscule total amount of food to do this. Signs that your body is having a stress event might be cold hands and feet, a sudden urge to urinate, frequent urination, a sudden crash in mood or energy levels, abnormalities in your pulse rate, a headache, nausea, a funky taste in your mouth or dry mouth, a loss of the pink color in your tongue – all kinds of things.

In terms of what kind of snack to eat, think back to one of the rules I mentioned earlier – eat a salty, carby snack. I tell people "the airlines got it right" when it comes to de-stressing foods and keeping passengers calm and at ease. A handful of salty pretzels or peanuts and a little cup of a sugary soft drink is a pretty good combination. Sugar, starch, salt, fat.

I like the dry, salty, carby convenience snacks for stress events. I have tried all kinds of things, from white sugar under the tongue to shots of maple syrup to a bite of fruit to dried fruit. And that helps. But without the salt it's just not as powerful. I like to see carbohydrates and salt combined to cover all bases. Foods like pretzels, potato or corn chips, Bugles (an old school snack food that I like a lot because it's cooked in coconut oil instead of vegetable oil like pretty much all other common snack foods), wasabi peas, cheese and crackers, dried fruit and cheese (especially dates), beef jerky with a little bit of something sweet, some pretzel M&M's, or a combination of a few things is all you really need. That may sound like a lot but I'm literally talking about 2-3 bites here, to lift you out of your slump and bridge the gap in between meals or whenever you need it – including before bed or in the middle of the night with the all too common 3-4am adrenaline surge.

In today's often chaotic environment, taking a break to have a meal has almost become old-fashioned. But it's reasonably practical to carry any number of these items with you and take some "medicine" when you need it. It works. It helps. And it's good to at least be paying a little bit of attention to what's going on in your physical body no matter what you are engaged in.

Snacks don't make up the bulk of anyone's diet, especially if you do truly stick to just having 2-3 bites when needed. So I wouldn't stress too much about what exactly you eat during a stress event. I actually believe that the more refined and rapidly-absorbed the food is, and the faster your stress system is deactivated, the better. There are actually advantages to many of the foods I just mentioned. But find out what you like, what works, and what you are comfortable with. Use it to keep your metabolism out of the gutter at all times.

If it seems too complicated, and your stress events are particularly strong and acute, you might consider keeping it really simple and making up a little baggy of a salt and sugar mix to carry with you. A small spoonful of this mixture dissolved directly under the tongue is a godsend for many. Since they typically use saline or sugar for placebos, this is guaranteed to at least trigger the placebo effect! I don't have a magic formula for what the ratio of sugar to salt should be in your mixture, but I would think 5:1 would be the minimum, and it will probably require a much higher ratio of sugar to salt to be palatable. Depends though, as during a severe crash many note pure salt tasting delicious. This does have, from my investigations thus far, a powerful medicinal effect when in need. If you're really in bad shape don't forget this one.

The salt and sugar mixture is an absolute must for nighttime stress events. For wakeups between 2-4 am, accompanied by a feeling of excess adrenaline circulating through your system (adrenaline peaks at this time), salt and sugar under the tongue is the only way to go. You don't want to be chewing anything, wandering around the house looking for food, opening the fridge and looking at bright lights when hoping to fall back asleep, and so forth. You want to remain as unstimulated as possible. Keep the sugar/salt mixture by the bedside for easy and thoughtless access until you stop having middle-of-the-night wakeups.

Also keep in mind that some of the symptoms of having overly-concentrated body fluids and overly-diluted body fluids have some overlap. In fact, the nutritional system that turned me onto all this in the first place preached adamantly that the symptoms of being "too high" or "too low" in terms of the concentration of the urine were virtually indistinguishable. I wouldn't go that far, but be alert to the fact that you may just need a few sips of water or some other drink, not necessarily a snack to return to normalcy. You will make mistakes on both ends of the hydration spectrum as you start toying around with this, but in time you will learn to easily differentiate between the need to drink vs. the need to snack

Circadian Rhythms

Damn, just when you thought you had mastered this whole concept I come throwing a curveball at you like this, talking about Hershiser Rhythms or some gobbledy-gook.

It's circadian, not Hershiser you douche. Circa means like, close or something. Dian means day. Circadian basically means "about a day." Circadian rhythms are the sequence of hormonal secretions that take place and repeat themselves about every 24 hours, give or take.

For example, in a normal guy you should see testosterone and cortisol peaking in the morning, among other hormones. In the evening you would see cortisol bottoming out and melatonin and growth hormone rising. In the middle of the night adrenaline peaks, roughly around that 4am window[3]. The typical

---

[3] I had a brief stint with New Age spirituality many years ago. One of my teachers said that "the energy for the new day arrives at 4am." Well, kinda.

peak in body temperature is 6-8pm, perhaps not the best time to be stuffing your face with salt and calorie-dense food. We'll discuss that concept later.

Anyway, I find these rhythms to be highly significant, as we are simply not the same person all day long. There seems to be great power in adjusting food and fluid intake to sort of smooth things out in a sense, from day to night. Most with mood disorders will note feeling anxiety, depression, or whatever their issue may be at a certain time of day consistently, but not at other times. Same with energy levels, desire to exercise, physical pain, sex drive, and lots of different things. People simply peak at certain times of day, and bottom out at other times of day.

But it's nice to be more even keel and consistent. Nobody wants to drag ass all day long and then finally come to life at 9pm and be wired until 2 in the morning, unless you are a stripper or something. Actually I should take that back. Having that pattern would probably do wonders for your social life.

And to achieve this even keel-ness, there is great power in slightly tweaking your food and beverage consumption based on your daily rhythms. The idea is to lift yourself up a little bit during the low part of the day, and then flatten the peak slightly. It seems as if our daily biorhythms function on a 24-hour wave, and

---

There may be a more logical explanation than cosmic waves being delivered by some elf-like stork from the 7th level of Astral light though. Adrenaline will definitely energize you, and I find 4am to be a consistent time to wake up frantic and not be able to return to sleep for those with a compromised metabolism.

anything that causes a greater peak or a greater trough apart from the midline creates instability. In other words, what goes up must come down, which is why you want to not only lift yourself up during your off hours, but actually reel in the height of your peak during the good half of the day.

This may not be making total sense, but it will as you keep reading, and as you start implementing and observing.

The most common or what I would call the typical pattern is to have cortisol peak in the morning, and thyroid peak in the early evening. Because of this, you really need a boost early in the day. Later in the day you're fine, and there's no reason to stuff your face with particularly calorie dense, warming types of meals. A lighter meal of soups, salads, fruit, lean meats, less added fat and salt, and what are otherwise the quintessential health foods is probably more appropriate.

One of the best indicators is to simply note what time of day your feet are most likely to get cold. The majority of people have the hardest time keeping their feet warm after breakfast, or early in the day in general – like around 10-11am. I, for example, have to eat my heaviest (most warming) meal of the day in the morning to keep my feet warm throughout an entire 24-hour day. I also typically need a mid-morning snack around 10am for extra insurance and a full lunch.

Once I've done that however, it's almost impossible for me to rid myself of those toasty warm hands and feet, even if I drink a considerable amount of fluids, and even if I eat absolutely nothing for dinner at all (although I do eat a regular full dinner, especially when I'm exercising a lot, just to get in adequate calories for recovery).

Others, however, don't have such a pattern. They may feel totally warm all morning and all afternoon and then, suddenly, a couple hours after dinner they start to feel freezing cold, urinate frequently, and prance off to bed with two pairs of socks just to keep their toes from turning purple in the night. A bigger dinner and a very warming late-night snack, such as a little salty popcorn and ice cream, eliminates this problem and keeps this person in more of a 24-hour long state of stability.

Others still don't notice much variation between day and night, but they still might notice a consistent 3pm crash in mood, energy, or the onset of coldness or a sudden strong urge to urinate. Becoming aware of this and eating a preemptive warming snack, BEFORE the crash happens, can often prevent it from ever occurring. Or you could just be noticing this effect because your breakfast was too light and cooling, which will cause you to have a tendency to feel more drowsy after lunch if that's the case. Generally the more time you spend in a cold state, the more drowsy and the more complete the shutdown of your nervous system is when you finally get a belly full of warming foods.

But that is getting more into what I wanted to save for the next interesting observation – what I call the overcompensation effect.

For now, what I want you to get out of this chapter is that there is a great deal of power when it comes to tweaking your meal schedule around to create greater physiological stability within.

Most will find that they feel and function better staggering their warming food intake towards the first half of the day, and ramping up the cooling food intake towards the second half of the day. But like I said, I've encountered many who don't fit that profile at all, and I certainly empower you to figure that out for yourself. For those who hate breakfast and feel turned off by it in the morning, this can usually be overcome pretty quickly. I find this to be a particularly problematic pattern for some people, as long-term attempts at dieting, trying to abstain from food as long as possible each day only to binge late at night is a well-ingrained and very self-deprecating relationship with food. This type of eating behavior is also tightly correlated with obesity. Breaking this pattern can be a real game changer.

Anyway, that's enough to introduce the concept. Next let's just look at what a few variations in eating throughout the day looks like.

Adjusting Meal Schedule and Structure

To better help you envision what I mean, although I certainly don't recommend measuring anything out or being a freak about it, here's what a typical day might look like for someone with a tendency to peak in the evening and feel a tendency towards cold feet mid-morning...

Breakfast: 2 buckwheat pancakes with bananas, syrup, and whipped cream, 2 eggs scrambled with lots of salty cheese, small juice
Snack: A few grapes, cheese and crackers
Lunch: 2 cheeseburgers, slice of apple pie, Coke
Snack: 1 peach
Late afternoon: Glass of water
Dinner: Vegetable beef soup, large salad with pears, glass of milk
Before bed: Small glass of water

It's important to remember that for some this would be way too many fluids. For others, not enough. It really depends on where you're at metabolically. Some people cannot drink any plain water at all to start, or even juice, but have to start out consuming very little fluids in addition to the water naturally bound in food. Sometimes just a small glass of milk or a soft drink with each meal is all one can handle. Over time fluid requirements increase.

Let's take a look at what a proper structure might be for someone who has an extremely low metabolic rate, and has a tendency to be cold all day and all night, urinating every hour or even more often than that, including several urinations before bed and needing to wake up and urinate multiple times during the night. This would be typical of someone recovering from a fitness competition, eating disorder, or anything that caused substantial weight loss including dieting. The issue here is just getting a lot of low-water, highly palatable and digestible dense calories in, and eating more frequently. Generally the stronger a person's health the longer he or she can go without food…

4am: Sugar and salt under the tongue to fall asleep after sudden wakeup
8am: Waffles with sugared strawberries, salted butter and syrup, sausage, homefries
10am: Pint of ice cream, potato chips
12pm: Cheeseburger and milkshake
3pm: Beef stir fry with small soft drink

6pm: Macaroni and cheese, small glass of whole milk, chocolate chip cookies
9pm: Popcorn and small soft drink
Right before bed: Ice cream sandwich

Let's look at another scenario, and sorry to shock you with some of the food selections if you're a health nut. The last one was an extreme example in need of extremely dense and palatable calories. I decided to use common foods and common meals here to help make it easier to conceptualize of these principles. Our next example might be someone who seems to feel fine all day, but has an evening crash, frequent urination, ice cold feet, and difficulty falling asleep...

8am: Breakfast cereal, 1 piece of fruit
10am: 1 Medjool date, glass of water
1pm: Fish stew, rice, salad, juice
6pm: 3 slices of veggie pizza, soft drink
10pm: Scoop of ice cream, handful of potato chips

Hopefully you are observing the patterns here. The idea is to simply stagger your most warming foods of the day towards the time of day you feel cold or flat. Then, by increasing fluid intake and eating more water rich foods as well as lightening up on the big S's, salt especially, you work on achieving a more cooling effect during the other half of the day.

As a last example, let's look at what a day in the life of someone who is pretty healthy and balanced might look like – sort of a healthy, sustainable long-term drink and diet pattern. Pay attention to how the cooling and warming substances are there together to maintain a balance between the two. Damn, I'm sounding like a Buddhist monk or something…

8am: Oatmeal with fruit, butter, sugar, 2 eggs with cheese, large juice
10am: Apples and cheese
1pm: Beef chili, sandwich, cornbread, strawberry milkshake, glass of water
2pm: Glass of water
4pm: 1 peach
6pm: Potato soup, large salad, 2 plums, glass of water
9pm: Glass of water

   With the last example you see a much higher water intake accompanying what is still a pretty high energy diet. A person with a strong metabolism typically needs to eat and drink a lot. A person with a low metabolism needs to eat a lot and drink very little. Who needs to eat very little and drink a lot? No one that I've come across yet. Maybe some starving guy that lives near the equator with no air conditioning. Who eats very little and drinks a lot? Fricking everybody these days – at least everybody that reads health books!!! That's why a book like this needs to exist. Hey, at least if you're going to be starving yourself of calories or carbs or something to try to lose some weight or whatever (which I don't condone), don't compulsively drink while you do it.

And this probably doesn't need to be mentioned, but I will mention it anyway to avoid any confusion…

DON'T FOLLOW ANY OF THE ABOVE EATING AND DRINKING SCHEDULES VERBATIM!!!

That's not why I wrote them up. They are merely to serve as a conceptual aid. You must not follow any kind of health recipe verbatim, or you will likely get yourself in serious trouble, especially when it comes to consuming measured amounts of salt, calories, and fluids with no regard to your biofeedback and instincts. Plus, every day is completely different as I've already alluded to. A crappy night's sleep can dramatically lower your "fluid tolerance" the following day, and increase your need for calorie dense foods and salt. So can stress, or exercise, or any number of different things. You have to be flexible. You have to listen to your body, not me or anyone else. All I'm doing is increasing your awareness so that you are better armed to do that successfully on your own.

The Overcompensation Effect

I don't know how to explain this without sounding a little weird. And seeing that the subject of this book is already a little weird compared to what most "health" books are about, I'm sure you're ready to toss me and my book into the looney bin. Well, I have to mention it though, because it's very interesting.

I think it's reasonable to say that many of our biological systems have an overcompensation tendency. Like when you try to force some weight off with a diet. You don't just return to the same level of body fat later. You surpass it. The body overcompensates for the shortage.

Or how about when you've had diarrhea for a couple days? You often get a little constipated when that subsides, or vice versa.

The same strange thing occurs with the body and all this fluid stuff, including the stress response itself. For example, if you wait a really, really long time to eat, get super outrageously hungry, and then pig out… your stress system overcompensates and shuts down completely. Your eyelids feel like they weigh a thousand pounds. At least most would note this tendency.

Or how about a time when you were strung out overworking and only sleeping 5 hours a night for a week or two? What happened when you got your first big 8-hour plus night? Did you get sick or feel hungover like you "overslept?" I think the "oversleep" coma comes from the adrenal glands basically going on vacation to compensate, maybe even overcompensate, for prolonged overwork.

Anyway, the overcompensation effect factors into the hot/cold, high-stress/low-stress, body fluid concentration equation. The overcompensation effect is the reason why I find stockpiling your foods towards what is your colder part of the day so vital.

Let me explain how it typically works in a normal person. Let's say that you are colder with a greater tendency to urinate frequently with low-concentration urine mid-morning. But it's your habit to only have a bunch of coffee in the morning (tons of fluids, no food), pick at a small lunch or maybe try to eat a "good," diet-ish kind of lunch (Coolio might refer to you as one of those "salad-eatin' bitches"), drink a bunch of water all day doing a stressful job, and then later in the evening you pig out on majorly dense calories with lots of salt, sugar, starch, and fat. What happens? You actually get uncomfortably hot and may even encounter some pronounced negative symptoms

— like restless legs, trouble sleeping, bad dreams, night sweats, irritability, uncomfortably hot hands and feet, headaches, chest pressure, heavy pulse, and others.

But eating a simple breakfast instead of fasting and avoiding the excess fluids and frequent urination during the morning hours will eliminate this reaction to a big night-time meal. Take it a step further by really emphasizing both breakfast and lunch and hydrating more in the second half of the day and you can stay much more even keel throughout a full 24-hour cycle.

So in a sense, overhydrating during the day and undereating can cause a state of dehydrating overcompensation in the evening.

Likewise, eating big in the evening when you are already warm and the concentration of your fluids are in the right zone, and your body will overcompensate the next day by becoming easily overhydrated.

It's weird I know, but getting your hands and feet too warm the night before can make them too cold the next day. Getting your body fluids too strong at night can make them too weak the next day. Balance Daniel-san!!! Okay, that's a really overused quote. You should be disappointed in me. At least I didn't say "You can't handle the truth!"

You'll notice if you look around long enough, hopefully you won't, that those practicing a fast-all-day, eat big at night type of regimen (a typical setup for many forms of the increasingly trendy "intermittent fasting") often report cold hands and feet during the day and signs of high adrenaline (wow dude, I'm like so focused and have so much energy and I'm not even hungry!). And then at night they talk about how all their veins are bursting out of their skin, and the extreme warmth they feel. This is a prime example of a massive unbalanced roller coaster ride happening on the inside. Maybe it's harmless. In my experience, it's not harmless at all and can prevent a sick person from consistently making progress towards better, more resilient health.

So one thing I tell people is that you shouldn't necessarily pig out all day long. This is fine when you're in a really extreme place and just need to pack on a bunch of fat to get your system working correctly again. But for the average person with just a little hill to climb, it can actually be counter-productive to eat big when you are already in the ideal metabolic state. It's better, when you're already in the right zone, to simply perpetuate that state by eating a good balance of cooling, water-rich foods and fluids along with your warming substances.

Instead, eat big and drink small when you need to concentrate your fluids. Eat light and drink more when you are already nice and warm in the hands and feet and feeling really solid. For some this will mean eating heavy during the day and light at night. For others this will mean eating lightly during the day and heavier at night. It's all about using this awareness to keep your body, and your cells, in a more stable state all the time. A "zone" you could call it.

Simple enough yes, but I thought it would be worthwhile to make you aware of this overcompensation effect. Awareness of course is the

repeating theme here. That's the point of this book –
to make you aware of something that wasn't at all on
your radar screen, but is easy and natural to do and can
be applied to just about any other eating paradigm –
including just the standard diet that is normal amongst
your friends and family. And that's the beauty I guess.
You don't have to do anything weird really. Just make
a few fine-tuned adjustments that can still have a
substantial effect on how your body functions and the
direction your health is moving in.

How Much Salt?

That is the question. And there's no real answer. It really depends. There are several routes you can take. One is that you can reduce your fluid consumption and keep your salt consumption the same. This seems pretty reasonable with the modern diet in general, because it doesn't seem to lack salt. Of course, as alluded to before, most people reading health books aren't necessarily eating a modern diet and modern foods and are often living off of smoothies and green juices and salads instead with 3 additional quarts of water on top of it – none of which have much salt at all. The fluid levels are off the charts.

I run into people like this all the time, and they typically crave salt like crazy. Adding lots of salty foods to the diet really helps. But without all the damn fluids and watery "health" foods that may be nothing shy of inappropriate if their metabolic rate is below normal, there really is no reason to go overboard with the salt.

So it's really up to you to personally determine whether it makes more sense to cut back your fluids or increase your salt. Some will need to do both. I tend to lean more towards cutting back the fluids because I do view the modern habit of having a drink or bottle in hand at all times as being compulsive and totally abnormal compared to the past – or compared to the rest of the animal kingdom for that matter. You won't see a cow having 58 sips of water during the day, even if she is grazing right next to a river. Those that I see clutching to a drink at all times remind me of Linus attached to his blanket all day. It's just weird. It's not quite right.

Plus, if you do add a lot of salt to your diet, which will increase your thirst and increase your need for fluids to dilute that salt, that could spell trouble if you are a soft drink junkie. For some, adding salt will probably just make them drink another two or three cans of soda. This may be inconsequential for some people, for others it may be quite a problem. Even with my lackadaisical approach to diet I still can't condone drinking two quarts of Mountain Dew a day. It's a poor nutritional investment despite any lack of ill consequences in the short-term.

So the answer is far from straightforward and simple. But ultimately let's take a look at the maximum and kind of work our way backwards.
The original research that yielded the mass prescription to drink "8, 8-ounce glasses of water a day," which was later revised to something like "drink half your body weight in fluid ounces each day" was based on total water consumption needs. So this has nothing to do

with how much water you drink, as water is in everything from pepperoni pizza to scrambled eggs. What this refers to is total fluid intake. Still, it's a crude measure as the lower a person's metabolism, the lower his or her fluid needs are, but we'll use it for conceptual purposes.

Let's say you weighed 200 pounds and thus needed 100 ounces of fluid each day – about 3 liters of total fluid. For that fluid to be "isotonic" by the medical industry's standards, which calls .9% saline "isotonic," you would need to take in 27 grams of salt with all that fluid. That certainly approaches what I would consider the maximum, although very hypertonic solutions of up to 7.5% salt have been used in extreme cases of shock and stuff like that.

While 27 grams of salt per day may seem extreme, as Americans consume roughly 9 grams per day, there are places in Asia where this much salt is consumed, and consumed by people that weigh less than 200 pounds. So it's not completely crazy to be throwing around numbers like this. I believe there are probably some severely hypothyroid people that could use a nice salt-loading phase to get out of seriously low places as well. In my experience, by far the most warming meals are those that contain 10 grams of salt or higher, so intakes up around 30 grams per day shouldn't be completely ruled out, especially when rebounding from something like an intense eating disorder, highly restrictive diet, or overzealous exercise program. Once again, the lower the metabolism the higher the need for salt. As metabolic rate increases, salt intake can begin to taper off, and probably will naturally as I find an increase in thirst and decrease in salt appetite to take place with increasing body heat.

As a reference, the National recommended intake for a typical adult is not to exceed 6 grams of salt per day. So we are talking about some pretty hefty amounts here. I can't help but to encourage some caution on behalf of anyone implementing some of the ideas in this book when it comes to going anywhere beyond 30 grams in a day. That seems a bit reckless to me.

Of course we still can't say that 30 grams per day is too much for everyone because salt intake in simple gram measurements doesn't account for the tremendous variability in size from person to person. If we are to consume "half our body weight in fluid ounces each day," and 9 grams of salt is in every 34 fluid ounces (1 liter) of "isotonic saline," then we have to figure the maximum to be roughly around 9 grams of salt per 68 pounds of person. This calculation would come out to be about 1 gram of salt for every 7.55 pounds of body weight. This puts the maximum salt intake at roughly 20 grams for a 150-pound person.

While this calculation probably has very little real-world usage, if you want to calculate your own theoretical max salt consumption, based arbitrarily on isotonic saline, body weight with no regard for body composition (how much of your weight is fat vs. muscle), and the status quo on daily fluid consumption, then you can do it by dividing your body weight in pounds by 7.55, or your body weight in kilograms divided by 3.43. Thus...

$$225 \text{ pounds} / 7.55 = 29.8 \text{ grams of salt}$$
$$100\text{kg} / 3.43 = 29.2 \text{ grams of salt}$$

Okay okay I'll stop! Give me a break. All this writing and writing and writing. Can't a guy squeeze a little math in once in a while? It feels good. I don't want to think that all those endless hours I spent playing Math Blasters on my Apple IIe was in vain. Let's leave it at this when it comes to your own personal salt intake...

The first is to be aware of both your salt and your fluid intake, in a rough sense. Don't necessarily track it or weigh and measure – this need not eclipse your life. But become salt and fluid aware, which is really all I'm seeking to get out of you by writing a book on this topic and bringing all this to your attention.

Fluids are great, and we need them to have extracellular fluid, build blood, and prevent our cells from shriveling up like little raisins. Dehydration is indeed an extreme stress. But consume a reasonable amount of fluids. If you are pursuing some kind of puritanical health food diet with lots of unrefined, high-water content foods, be even more reasonable with your added beverages.

In addition to that, add the appropriate amount of salt. This should really be guided primarily by...

• Taste

• Total water consumption

In general, the higher the total water consumption from all sources, the higher the salt needs. Things like exercise on a hot day cause us to sweat, and we lose lots of salty water. We need to replace this salty water by taking in more salt and more fluids. This should be factored in as well.

And, just like our thirst being the best dictator of our fluid needs under normal circumstances (extreme physiological stress will cause thirst to become inappropriately high), our natural tastes and desires are a decent roadmap to our accompanying salt needs. Add salt and salty condiments like soy sauce until the taste is just to your liking, and be sure to add a salty component to each meal and snack. It doesn't always take an astronomical amount to satisfy our salt desires, especially if you are consuming a reasonable amount of fluids.

Somewhere between the moderate 6 grams and turning Japanese at 30 grams or higher, you will hopefully find a balance. The amount will change too. You may very well start off needing and craving very large amounts before it tapers off after a few days or weeks. You may feel great as your metabolism rises and you start exercising a lot and sweating three times as much as normal, and your salt needs might steadily increase. There's really no way to definitively know such a thing with certainty, and that's part of the beauty of this type of book. It encourages mindfulness and a few basic understandings and tips on how to better interpret our body's signals, but aside from that leads one away from trying to intellectualize what the body needs. Many just need their brains to shut up and listen to be guided back to a balanced, healthy state.

Likewise, your salt needs may vary during the day depending on your natural rhythms. Like I discussed earlier, consuming a higher salt to fluid ratio may be great during the morning hours when most people have a stronger tendency to feel colder with higher stress hormone exposure. Then this can be flip-flopped in the early evening when body temperature rises and you actually need the cooling effects of more fluids and less salt.

As a final tip on the salt issue, it seems like salt consumption is automatically higher when one consumes a heavier diet composed more of meats and starches. Think of steak and potatoes for example, both of which take on a very large amount of salt before they taste absolutely mwah! I think problems often arise when there is too great of a departure from this template, and people start relying more and more on convenience foods, bagels, ice cream, candy, fruit, little snacks, and so forth. You simply don't consume much salt when you rely on convenience foods as more of your staples, departing from a more traditional 3 squares a day meal template. Sure, those foods are fine, but as a snack that is an afterthought to a meal – not eclipsing the hearty and satisfying meals themselves.

So what I'm saying, simply, is to eat real meals with traditional salty components such as a big starchy centerpiece and a small portion of meat, fish, eggs, or dairy products – all seasoned with salt to the point where the flavors pop. Don't get in the habit of relying solely on quickie foods like bagels, Pop Tarts, breakfast cereal, toast, fruit, smoothies, and other increasingly popular on-the-go type of foods. From there just let your natural salt meter dictate how salty those foods should be.

And of course no chapter on salt would be complete without a little discussion on what type of salt a person should use, as I'm sure many reading this have been wondering since the beginning. Well, any kind will do in my experience. Salt is salt. There is an increasing trend towards the use of sea salt in health circles. Sea salt does have trace minerals and is more "natural." Ultimately I found the "natural" paradigm to be extremely limiting and sort of a wild goose chase that disregards fact in pursuit of a philosophy. I don't recommend blindly being a naturalist with religiosity as I once did. I basically just ended up starving and freezing my ass off in the Wilderness on a diet of mostly trout with every metabolic sign in complete shutdown.

Currently I think of sea salt, natural as it may be, as salt with toxic sea sludge attached. Well, I wouldn't go that far, but it's probably best not to think in one narrow line of thinking where sea salt should be worshipped and all other salt should be neurotically avoided. I eat Morton's Canning and Pickling salt. It has a good, pure, salt flavor. It's not like that nasty, chemical-flavored iodized table salt stuff. And it's better than Kosher salt too.

And I really enjoy soy sauce a lot. It's probably best to get higher quality soy sauce that is traditionally fermented using soybeans (true Tamari) rather than the stuff that is made from hydrolyzed soy protein and wheat – like cheap store-bought Kikkoman swill. Damn it tastes good though! Like crack! While we're on the salty soy condiment kick, miso is damn fine too. The Japanese definitely know how to do salt right.

Alright, enjoy your salt. Don't believe the hype about how it's going to make your blood pressure skyrocket and your kidneys explode. It's actually more likely to deactivate the renin-angiotensin system, build blood volume, and ultimately normalize your blood pressure amongst other de-stressing functions. Just remember the signs that you've overdone it that I mentioned earlier and you'll be fine.

What to Drink?

I think the most reasonable way to set up this chapter is to just break down a bunch of common drinks and then discuss the pros and cons of each. That way we can look at some of the properties of certain beverages in greater detail – going through them one by one. In a general sense, the most important thing of all is that you are drinking because you are motivated by genuine thirst – not hunger, or being hot or cold, or boredom, or to obtain a drug like aspartame, alcohol, or caffeine. If you do drink for motivations other than thirst, as we all do at times in our modern beverage-centric social scene,[4] at least chase it with some high-octane food. Without further ado…

---

[4] How weird is that? I mean, we are expected to hang out and have drinks at night with friends, and meet friends during the day for coffee or tea. When I rule the world the drinks have gotta go and everyone will gather around a big pile of fries cooked in coconut oil. And then get it on.

Water – Water is fine to drink, in general. But it depends entirely on where a person is metabolically. If you have severe problems with frequent urination and display some of the major signs and symptoms that are associated with diluted body fluids and a very low metabolic rate – such as being very cold, dry mouth, dizziness, blurred vision, headaches, migraines, mood instability, insomnia, anxiety, dry skin, and many others… I find plain water to be counterproductive starting out. Someday you may be able to drink water as your primary beverage. But be open to the idea that a sugar-rich, or better yet, a salt and sugar-rich beverage might be right for you as you work your way towards normalcy.

Otherwise water is best consumed in small amounts by itself, only to satisfy thirst of course, or with food so that it is packaged with electrolytes and carbohydrates – and thus much less likely to aggravate problems and "wash you out" as I call it.

I drink some water most days – some days consuming well over a liter. Still, I recommend erring on the side of underconsumption of plain water rather than overconsumption unless you are truly subjecting yourself to extreme heat and exertion. But even if you are doing that, you will still fare better with salt and sugar-rich fluids that approximate lost sweat. A good friend of mine actually almost lost his life trying to stay hydrated while doing grueling outdoor exercise by consuming a couple gallons of plain water throughout the day. He was suffering from severe hyponatremia, the most frequent cause of death and illness from

marathon runners and other water-chugging extremists.
He drinks Gatorade now, and eats plenty of food with
his fluid consumption so as not to consume too many
fluids all by themselves. Problem solved.

Mineral Water – Mineral water has some minerals in
it, and those are helpful, but ultimately the electrolyte
content is negligible. Mineral water should therefore be
treated more like water and consumed with caution by
those with good metabolic health and largely avoided
by those in much weaker shape.

Fruit Juice – Fruit juice seems like a great alternative
to water, and in some cases it is. Ultimately I suffered
from a lot of cognitive dissonance at first when many
would fare really well on nutritionally bankrupt soft
drinks yet have all their symptoms aggravated by fruit
juice. It became obvious later that fruit juice, really low
in sodium but extremely high in potassium, was to
blame for this. In terms of electrolytes, fruit juice is
really a mismatch with our extracellular fluid. While it's
important to get potassium in the diet, that potassium
should really be counterbalanced with sodium for those
in an impaired state. You often see those who discuss
the topic of adrenal fatigue steering people towards salt
and away from potassium, and this may be valid.

I recommend consuming fruit juice in moderation
with meals. If you are going to drink it alone without
any other fluids, it is sometimes more stabilizing to
dilute it with water by at least 50% and add a
considerable amount of salt to liken it to a true

rehydration formula – something like Pedialyte or Rehydran-N, which are popular rehydration formulas used by entities like the World Health Organization to rehydrate children with dysentery. http://drugbase.org/drugs/drug_details.php?drugid=172 2 These have saved as many lives as just about any drug ever created with the exception of perhaps antibiotics. And the combination of sugar, sodium, the other electrolytes in fruit juice such as potassium and magnesium – makes diluted fruit juice with added salt a great drink with hard exercise as sweat replacement.

Ultimately the sugar in fruit juice is very therapeutic to someone in need of concentrating body fluids, but the total quantity of juice taken in should be relatively small. I don't think it should be a major portion of your fluid intake I guess I should say, or at least not consumed to excess like it often is in other pro-metabolism programs.

As a final word on fruit juice, lumping all fruit juices together is pretty foolish. Each fruit and each fruit juice is different in terms of its amount of potassium and the type, quantity, and proportion of different types of sugars. For example, grape juice and apple juice is much lower than orange juice in the potassium category. So experiment freely and don't necessarily group all fruit juices together as if they are the same. Some fruit juices may make you feel completely different than another variety.

Coconut water – Coconut water, which is becoming an increasingly trendy alternative to soft drinks and plain water, should be treated a lot like other fruit juices. It has some sodium and is well-known for having "electrolytes," but I hear frequently that it can make people feel pretty miserable after drinking it, and they aren't sure why. I would assume much of it has to do with the high ratio of potassium to sodium. Once again, potassium is sort of the polar opposite of sodium – the primary electrolyte found in extracellular fluid. The poorer metabolic shape a person is in, usually the more sodium they need in proportion to potassium.

Milk – Milk is usually a superb, warming, metabolism-stimulating beverage. It has some sodium in it, and is generally one of the most mineral-dense foods on earth, but the real key seems to be the fat in milk. The higher the fat content of a dairy product, generally the more warming it is. A liter of fat free skim milk is very cooling on one end of the spectrum. On the other end of the spectrum, drinking sweetened half and half (a 50:50 mixture of milk and cream) is like pouring ice cream down your throat and is extremely warming. It's also exorbitantly freaking delicious. A couple teaspoons of blackstrap molasses or maple syrup in a cup of half and half is an extremely warming addition to any meal, and is very warming consumed all by itself unlike almost any other beverage.

For someone in a low metabolic state, there is hardly any more appropriate substitution for water than whole milk or, even better, half and half. Adding a little bit of extra salt and sugar to milk or half and half makes these extremely thermogenic compared to other beverages. But even whole milk with added sugar and salt can still be cooling in excess if you take the total consumption too far. It's still not something that you should force down your throat, but something to have a small cup of when thirsty.

If you notice a very pronounced cooling effect when consuming milk, half and half, or even ice cream – that lasts beyond the 20-30 minutes it takes for your body to heat up the cold fluid (assuming you are consuming it cold – heating up half and half or whole milk is awesome by the way), you may have a mild allergy to it. That doesn't mean that you have to live with that forever. I see people overcome food allergies and intolerances regularly as overall health improves. But that may be what is setting off the stress system and making the hands and feet feel very chilled. It may be something that you need to temporarily avoid until the metabolic rate improves. I point this out as yet another reminder that nothing is universally warming or cooling. It's up to you to figure that out for yourself.

Sports Drinks – Sports drinks are great in theory. There are a few things that I like about them, and a few things that I don't like. Overall, they are a better choice than soft drinks and often fruit juice too (although there are dozens of types of fruit juices, and each is different). They contain more salt, less sugar, no caffeine, and the sugar used in them is typically a 2:1 glucose to fructose blend which usually doesn't include reliance on high-fructose corn syrup. Not that I am some kind of anti high-fructose corn syrup Nazi – I still consume some products that contain it. But overall sucrose from cane sugar seems a better choice. It tastes better and leaves no aftertaste either like HFCS often does.

The problem with sports drinks is that, in order to be profitable, the formula is far from being ideal from a hydration standpoint, and is more ideal from a taste perspective. Compared to what is ideal for hydration, there is a lot more sugar and a lot less salt. People don't necessarily want to drink something that tastes salty and isn't that sweet. This was one ironic finding when it came to rehydration formulations for people who were sick or starving in developing countries – as the scientists tweaked the formula for better performance (more salt, less sugar), usage of it declined and they were faced with a tough decision.

Anyway, sports drinks are not a bad choice. You may come to prefer just making your own blend of salty, diluted fruit juice though until you are able to drink plain water without any negative recourse.

Coffee – Coffee is like water on steroids, making people crash and become even more diluted it seems. It's a tough topic too because most people don't drink coffee because they are thirsty, which overall is my biggest issue with coffee. What I recommend is really going heavy on the half and half – maybe even making or ordering something like a breve latte, which is made with half and half instead of milk. Half and half functions more like a warming food than a cooling beverage, so it really helps to counteract the coffee.

Adding plenty of sugar and even a little salt (much tastier than it sounds) can actually make for quite a warming drink. I don't think many people will need to avoid coffee to have good health. But don't drink it in excess and balance it out properly with the warming substances – fat, sugar, and salt. At least drink it with food if you can't manage to do that.

Tea – I could have pretty much copied and pasted the coffee section into here. Drink your tea actually brewed in hot milk or half and half with added sugar and salt (like a Chai). It too can be a very warming beverage instead of something that keeps people washed out all day as they keep hitting cup after cup.

Soy Milk – Don't even touch that shit. Warming or not doesn't matter. It is the devil haha. I practically gave myself IBS drinking tons of that in my 20's. Soy requires lengthy fermentation to be truly edible. Miso, tamari, natto – fine. Soy milk? Fuhgeddaboudit! If you do feel like you need some kind of "milk substitute" the best option is probably rice milk. But the stuff is like water and is very cooling. A bowl of cereal with rice milk in the morning isn't exactly going to get your toes cooking. So only small amounts. Or eat that bowl of cereal with a big side of salty fried potatoes. Don't forget coconut milk either. It's not really a drink or a milk substitute, but writing this section made me think about it and it's super warming.

Soft Drinks – Well, soft drinks are better than water for some people. I will be totally upfront and honest about that. They can even be better than fruit juice or trying to create some kind of super fruit-juice based sports drink with added salt. That may be hard to accept if you are a health nerd or have been swept away by the fructose paranoia that has taken the world by storm in recent years. I can relate. I've been there too. But it's not a bad option for people in bad shape. Replacing a gallon-a-day water habit with a few cans of straight up Coca Cola can be the primary difference between being healthy and being unhealthy. Of course, you don't have to drink soda just to eliminate compulsive water drinking. You can still drink water, just less. But even small amounts of water are flat-out harmful to someone in a truly compromised state.

On the flip side, some people compulsively drink sodas beyond physiological thirst because they taste good and have caffeine. For some, switching over to drinking boring ol' water eliminates the overconsumption of fluids.

So I guess if you are drinking soft drinks and feeling cold switch to water. If you are drinking water and feeling cold, switch to soft drinks! I'm actually not totally joking. Maybe 57% joking, 38% serious and 5% confused and disoriented.

Diet Sodas – Like full-sugared soft drinks when it comes to the dangers of compulsive overdrinking… but diet drinks are more cooling and more seductive in the addictive department. As mentioned earlier, aspartame, the sweetener in most commercial diet drinks, has many side effects that are identical to the side effects of excess fluid consumption – blurred vision, headaches, migraines, seizures, and so on… http://www.naturalnews.com/035242_aspartame_side_e ffects_neurological.html

I can't say for sure, but I suspect that most cases of these side effects when it comes to diet drink consumption come from excess fluid consumption. Many who drink diet drinks consume astronomical amounts of them in my observation, perhaps because they are viewed as "free calories." Of course, someone drinking a diet drink is also very likely to be consciously trying to restrict food intake, engaged in disordered eating behavior like starving and binging, and otherwise making themselves more sensitive to excess fluid consumption. Bad combination.

Anyway, even plain water is a far better choice than diet drinks.

Fermented Beverages – There is a lot of health propaganda given to fermented beverages. I don't think they are going to cause a repopulation of the bacteria in your digestive tract, nor do I think they will magically cure you of cancer or anything else. BUT, most fermented beverages like kefir, kvass, ginger beer, and kombucha are still great drinks. I don't have much negative to say about them other than the fact that commercial varieties of things like kombucha are criminally overpriced. They have a good balance of sugar and water and can outperform plain water in many cases, so you should be able to drink them in the right quantity with no ill effect.

Vegetable Juice – Vegetable juice like the commercial V-8, a super salty concoction with vegetable juice is probably a great overall drink. In writing this I kind of feel like a dummy for having not consumed it myself while playing around with this concept over the past year and a half. Even better might be to consume your own fresh vegetable juice concoction with added salt. Vegetables are high in potassium so it's probably best to counterbalance it with salt or food.

Just don't get too carried away with vegetable juice, especially if you are juicing raw cruciferous vegetables like kale or cabbage. They contain substances that are very harmful to the thyroid, especially when consumed uncooked. Raw vegetables in general have some potent anti-nutrients that are harmful to the body when consumed in large quantities. Stuff like spinach is very high in oxalic acid. So are beet greens and other nasty things that often find their way into people's juicers. Even beta carotene found in especially high amounts in carrots can be problematic in excess. So when you do consume vegetable juices, do it in moderation as a small supplement to an otherwise decent diet. Just because vegetable juice is nutritious does not mean the more you consume the healthier you will be.

Beer and Wine – Beer and wine, as well as mixed drinks, are what I consider to be the high-water alcoholic beverages. Although I rarely drink alcohol

myself, I would never expect someone to just give up
drinking alcohol completely for health reasons. Life is
too short, and it's usually not necessary to completely
give up alcohol to function at a high level. But when
drinking these high-water drinks in order to obtain
alcohol, which of course has absolutely nothing to do
with physiological thirst, it doesn't take too much extra
to get a person with a weakened system into serious
trouble.

If you are the type of person who has to start
running to the bathroom every 10 minutes with a very
strong urge to urinate after only one beer, be careful.
You can counteract this effect of alcoholic beverage
consumption by eating a heavy meal with your drinks –
preferably before, and then continuing to snack on dry,
salty bar food like chips, nachos, and pretzels
throughout the evening. The high carbohydrate and
salt intake from dry foods is a great way to have a night
of drinking with much less negative recourse the
following day.

A better option for someone who is more sensitive
might be to have a few shots of hard alcohol instead to
limit the risk of consuming too many fluids. That is
certainly a smarter strategy if there is no food to be
found wherever you are enjoying some drinks.

And yes, I know that alcohol makes you feel warm
in the hands and feet. That's because it does relax the
nervous system. I have even considered that small
amounts of alcohol here and there may be highly
medicinal in that regard. Ultimately I like to see people

getting that effect from food, from sleep, and from relaxing activities if possible, not drugs.

Anyway, that's all I have to discuss on specific fluids. Really not much more to say other than to remind you once more that the real danger with fluids of any kind is consuming those fluids beyond physiological thirst. But I'm sure you've gotten that by now. Please don't get your panties in a wad about me not coming out and chastising soft drinks or "x" thing that you think is poisoning all the people in the world. This book is not about that, and keeping your cells producing energy properly, your stress system quieted down – these measures represent big physiological changes that are much greater than whether you choose to drink coconut water instead of Pepsi. I hope that you can grasp that concept and not mentally tune me out as I did to other health writers with similar messages in the early days of my own health exploration.

Alright kids. Moving on…

Exercise

E xercise influences all this fluid crap in some very
noticeable ways too. In general, exercise is very
warming and puts your body into a much higher
metabolic state WHILE you do it and maybe for a
while after. But ultimately I have rarely seen exercise
translate to a higher resting metabolic rate and body
temperature. That doesn't mean you shouldn't exercise
or that it is a waste of time. It's not. Physical activity,
done by a healthy person in the right amount with
proper rest and recovery will usually just make him or
her feel happier and healthier with a more impressive
physique.

In the extracellular fluid department, exercise seems
to soak up a bunch of fluids into the muscle cells.
Doing some hard weightlifting for example will really
increase your thirst and threshold for fluids. No it's
not just the sweating from the activity itself. You can
sweat a liter and have to drink two it seems like to me,

and this increased water in the cell actually promotes muscle growth. Many successful bodybuilders swear by drinking copious amounts of water, and there is probably a great deal of validity to it. What you don't hear is that this stimulator of muscle growth – extra water in the cell, actually lowers cellular metabolic rate.

Anyway, I won't go into that too much. This isn't a book about muscle growth or even metabolic rate specifically – although that's obviously a keen focus of mine in all the books I have written. What I wanted to say about exercise is something like this…

If you exercise too hard, too long, or too frequently it can indeed have a net-diluting effect on your system as a whole. If I were to say, exercise really hard doing some circuit training for 5-6 days in a row, by the end of that week I would start having strange episodes of frequent urination. I actually use this as a gauge to determine how much is too much in the exercise department.

I would also say not to get too swept away by the warming effects of exercise. A good exercise session may keep you from urinating frequently for the rest of the day that you've done it, with toasty hands and feet and a general feeling of well-being. But if you pay attention, you'll notice that all is not well. When you take a day or two off you may notice feeling colder than normal, peeing more than normal, and having more clear urine than normal.

Take a whole week off from a hard exercise routine and just do light activities and you may notice feeling really warm and not peeing very frequently by the end of that week, even though at first you felt worse.

What I'm getting at is that you too, once you become more aware of urine concentration, the warmth of your hands and feet, achieving the warming effect from food, and so on, will notice that exercise has an effect. It is common to think that exercise is all warming and be encouraged to "just do it" every day. The "theory" that you start to develop after noticing this effect is only reinforced when a day without exercise causes you to feel flat, tired, cold, and "pissy."

This observation can be somewhat dangerous and misleading because in actuality you wouldn't feel cold and pissy on your days off if you weren't overdoing it. If you weren't doing any formal exercise you might be radiating massive body heat all the time. In general you don't want to become "dependent" on exercise to make you warm. You want to be able to generate great body heat with excellent circulation to the extremities without having to hit the gym or even walk around the block. Nothing wrong with those things, but there's certainly no shortage of overtraining going on in the health world.

It's also important to know that you don't have to really do much hard exercise to make significant changes to your physique – or at least to get the hormonal benefits from it. You can lift weights for 15 minutes a week and still get stronger every single week if your program is progress-oriented. You can improve cardiopulmonary output by doing some sprint intervals or something similar for about the same amount of time and frequency as well. What I'm getting at is that you can get stronger, faster, and more in-shape doing very little. The majority of people are either getting nowhere because they are doing nothing, or doing a lot and still not improving much because the element of progress isn't worked into their physical activity.

A smart, sustainable, progress-oriented approach (increasing weight or speed or overall intensity via shorter recovery periods) that yields improvements every single week can be designed and performed by just about anyone. Keep up with it for many years on a consistent basis, with steady progress, and you can get all the benefits of exercise with much less wear and tear on your system – you know, that wear and tear and physical and mental strain that has never allowed you to consistently do anything exercise-wise for more than a few months before reaching burnout.

Anyway, I hope to write at much greater length about this topic in the future, but this is obviously getting off topic. Just know that too much exercise can interfere with your ability to produce a great deal of body heat at rest. Don't become dependent on it to keep your hands and feet warm. Doing too much of it may actually be keeping you from feeling warm and toasty when you aren't doing it!

Disorders Most Likely to Be Affected

I've pretty much gotten across the concept. Now let's quickly look at exactly who is most likely to notice a significant change by playing around with it — "it" being the Eat for Heat concept you perv!

At the risk of sounding redundant, a really metabolically healthy person can drink a gallon of water a day and not experience any negative recourse at all. Likewise, a really metabolically healthy person could probably go a little low on calories, exercise a lot, and eat a low salt or low-carb diet with all this water and feel hardly any negative effects. But this type of person is becoming increasingly rare in my experience.

Thus, the person that is most likely to gain from more mindful management of the amount of elements such as carbohydrates, calories, and salt in proportion to fluid intake will be someone in a weakened metabolic condition. By weakened metabolic condition

I don't necessarily mean someone that has been diagnosed with actual hypothyroidism, although someone formally classified as "hypothyroid" will be very likely to experience improvement. Someone in a weakened metabolic condition can include all kinds of people – those with a naturally low metabolic rate, chronic dieters, someone who has recently undergone a major stress in life, those that are fanatical about eating the perfect diet including former low-carbers, vegans, raw foodists, etc., overexercisers, those that have recently lost weight, bulimics and anorexics, women having metabolic problems during or after pregnancy, hardgainers or those with low muscle mass, the elderly… and of course anyone suffering from a chronic illness (including chronic infections), most of which are highly influenced by the rate of cellular energy metabolism.

Those would be some of the general things that would predispose someone to a weakened metabolic condition. There are others, including some that I probably haven't even discovered yet.

Here are some more specific conditions and disorders that have a high likelihood of at least being improved by mastering body fluid concentration and increasing body temperature, if not eradicated or tightly controlled by it…

- Hypogonadism
- Dry skin
- Food sensitivities

- Raynaud's Syndrome
- Blurred vision
- Heart Palpitations
- Headaches and Migraines
- Seizures
- Premenstrual syndrome
- Constipation
- Chronic bacterial infection
- Brittle nails and hair
- Low sex drive
- Erectile dysfunction
- Tooth sensitivity
- Insomnia
- Chronic Fatigue Syndrome
- Anxiety/Panic attacks
- Depression
- Weight gain on low-calorie diet
- Infertility
- Hypertension
- Preeclampsia
- Morning sickness
- Poor milk quality and quantity
- Heavy or light periods
- Amenorrhea
- Dry mouth
- Inability to sweat
- Cold intolerance

- Nocturia and bedwetting
- Polyuria
- Tendency towards allergy and autoimmunity
- Nightmares or night terrors
- Hair loss
- Restless Leg Syndrome
- Breast underdevelopment
- Difficulty swallowing
- Poor appetite
- Low platelet count
- Low white blood cell count
- High cholesterol – especially high LDL/low HDL pattern
- High triglycerides
- Anemia
- Diabetes complications

There are many others. This list is not meant to be exhaustive. Any symptoms relating to hypothyroidism or a reduced metabolic rate apply, and this list is endless. As I often point out in interviews, one popular author on the subject of hypothyroidism has a chapter on symptoms that spans 85 pages!

Any symptoms related to hyponatremia also can be controlled, and those symptoms are both physical and psychological. It's been quite amazing to me to actually witness how many people are truly suffering from symptoms related to it, often caused directly by something they are doing to improve their health somehow (like drink a set amount of water, drink a bunch of vegetable juice, eat a low salt diet, etc.).

Those who don't suffer from anything acute enough to call a "symptom" or a "disease" still stand to gain some general increases in well-being, sleep quality, mood stability, sexual performance, enhanced immunity, and so on.

But if you do have some of the above-listed conditions, or a collection of some of those symptoms, you do owe it to yourself to apply this concept or methodology or whatever you wanna call it as a stand-alone or complementary therapy to what you're already doing. Over the years, I have communicated with someone with all of the above conditions at some point in time, and I've seen every item on that list improve or disappear in conjunction with an increase in core body temperature. That's no 100% guarantee. I don't wanna blow any smoke here. I've seen someone fail to overcome most of the items on that list as well. Nothing is foolproof. But odds are good you can see improvements in any one of those areas as you undergo a general health increase represented by better energy production.

FAQ

I have a history of urinary tract infections that I have dealt with primarily by drinking a ton of fluids. Is it wise for me to really follow this program? Am I at risk for developing UTI's again?

I don't think so. You certainly wouldn't want to take it to extremes or risk dehydration, as I do think more concentrated urine is indeed more aggravating to inflamed tissue in the urinary tract. But increasing body heat, body temperature, and thus metabolic rate is synonymous with an enhanced immune system. Overcoming chronic infections is very common with an increase in body heat generation and may very well rid you of your sensitivity to develop these infections in the first place.

Can this work on a low-carb diet?

In my experience a low-carb diet can be very metabolically-suppressive regardless of fluid and salt intake. The glucose seems necessary in order to take advantage of the salt itself, and there are known glucose transporters involved in the process, which is why rehydration drinks always contain glucose. I don't know what the minimum amount of carbohydrate would be to get the warming effect, but this is likely a matter that you will have to figure out for yourself via self-experimentation.

Won't this cause high-blood pressure if I eat more salt and drink less water?

Salt being the root cause of high blood pressure is a common fallacy. While I wouldn't blindly follow anything without making sure something like blood pressure isn't flying off the charts, I do think you'll discover that having more concentrated body fluids generally lends itself to having a deactivated stress system, and this deactivation of the stress system can normalize blood pressure, not make it go higher.

At first drinking less and eating more made me feel better. Now drinking more water makes my symptoms go away. Why is that?

Many symptoms that people experience on a day-to-day basis are from an activation of the stress system. The stress system can be activated by being overhydrated or dehydrated. As metabolism rises you actually need to drink more fluids, so what works in the beginning does not continue to work. As your body changes, your need for food and fluids changes with it. Do not cling to one "medicine." Certain formulas are only helpful in a certain metabolic state, and can actually be harmful in a different metabolic state. So you have to be alert to your changing body and make the necessary minor adjustments, most of them coming intuitively as appetite and thirst usually change when your metabolism changes.

Won't I get fat doing this?

People with a low metabolic rate are sometimes, but not always more prone to fat gain. As body temperature rises from say, 96 degrees F to 98 degrees F you may notice some gains in body fat. I would invest more time and energy into becoming fat-proof in a sense, being able to eat what you want, when you want without having to worry about accumulating fat. That's an empowering place to be, and if you had continued to forcefully starve yourself somehow by restricting your diet you probably would have gained that fat over time anyway. I say to hurry up and gain the fat so you can get your health back and stop gaining fat. A large percentage end up with a net gain of muscle mass and loss of body fat over time by eating for heat, and following the high body temperature where it leads you – basically the mirror opposite of yo-yo dieting, which makes your muscle mass become smaller and smaller while body fat levels climb higher and higher after each round. Your level of arousal for "fattening" foods decreases over time and desire and threshold for physical activity increases as well. Eating less and exercising more is the unconscious result of this approach. This is effectively a permanent way out of the conscious "eat less, exercise more" rat trap for those with the courage and the patience to see it through.

What about all the warm people that are sick or obese?

One indicator of body heat, such as the feeling of being hot, is not enough to gauge all that's going on inside. It's becoming increasingly well-known that despite often feeling warm, core body temperature is significantly reduced in the obese. A study of obese dogs revealed a very tight connection between reduced body temperature and obesity. The lower the body temperature, the more obese the dog. The same is generally true for humans, even amongst obese people who sweat constantly and have excessively hot hands and feet – often a result of having all that body fat creating the feeling of excess warmth. By the same token, we often feel cold when we have a fever or elevated temperature. Feeling warm, in and of itself, does not mean that metabolism is at its peak. It's just one indicator, and those that are feeling warm should still check body temperature to see if it is reduced, then take steps to increase core temperature the same as someone who feels chilly all the time.

Why are people looking to lose weight told to drink so much water?

Drinking cold water causes your body to burn extra calories to heat that water up. Water contains no calories and drinking lots of it reduces thirst for high-calorie beverages. Replacing soft drinks with water spontaneously reduces calorie consumption dramatically and can lead to weight loss in the short-term. Drinking lots of water can reduce appetite. These are all tricks to increase the level of starvation induced by diets, or to make the starvation more comfortable. This is not good for you nor does it mean you will succeed long-term with your weight loss just because it comes off more easily for the first few months. The "eat less, burn more" approach to weight loss has been proven endlessly to be ineffective long-term, and even counterproductive. But no one wants to believe it. They instead want to focus on the elusive first few months of dieting as if it is proof of an effective approach. It's not. There are other ways. There is a path of least resistance and self-starvation coupled with unwanted exercise and excessive water-chugging is not it.

What about bath water or swimming pools? Does that affect our body fluids?

It seems to a little bit, yes. While I wouldn't go out of your way to avoid baths, showers, swimming pools, hot tubs, and ponds – it might at least be worth taking a look into how really lengthy exposure to very hypotonic fluids impacts you (such as spending an entire hour in a swimming pool). If it is causing you significant problems, I would recommend taking warm baths in heavily-salted water, which could not only help you avoid the negatives but reverse that completely and make you feel even better.

Can taking in a bunch of water with colonics or enemas dilute your body fluids and cause hyponatremia and a drop in body temperature?

Yes, absolutely. Count on it.

I feel more tired doing this? What am I doing wrong?

Well you may be overdoing it a little bit on the food and salt, and getting too carried away with avoiding fluids. But I wouldn't be overly quick to assume that feeling tired is a sign of distress. Often feeling very tired and fatigued is a sign that the adrenals are finally taking a much needed break. I find spending time in a fatigued, but relaxed state, eating and sleeping a lot for many weeks even, can be one of the most therapeutic things a person can do. Sometimes feeling tired is simply retribution for having taxed your body too hard with diets, stress, lack of sleep, or a combination of things.

My mouth is dry all the time and I'm really thirsty! But if I obey that and drink as much as I want I'm cold and peeing all the time and having problems. What should I do?

Dry mouth is a symptom of the stress response being activated. It is officially a symptom of water intoxication and hyponatremia. It can be very misleading and is not genuine thirst. Eating calorie-dense foods with a lot of salt and choosing beverages with added sugar in place of water or tea is a good starting point for eliminating the dry mouth. As your system relaxes the dry mouth should subside. Be careful about drinking plain water until you feel confident you have distanced yourself from the dry mouth tendency.

I feel really hot – I'm even sweating at room temperature. But my hands and feet are still cold to the touch. What does that mean?

The stress system is likely still overly active. Adrenaline actually can make us feel quite hot. Weight loss pills chock full of stimulants are called "thermogenics" because they stimulate adrenal hormones, which in turn generate body heat. The coldness of the hands and feet is more revealing in this circumstance, and you should continue to "eat for heat" in terms of getting that stress system deactivated and feeling warm blood rush into the hands and toes.

Tools

I wouldn't recommend jumping right into obsessively using a thermometer to track changes in body temperature. Rely primarily on the feeling of relaxed, happy, calm, heat radiating all throughout your body all the way out to the tip of your toes. This is a great indicator of whether you have achieved the net warming effect of eating after ingesting food and/or fluids.

If you are still having trouble figuring things out, a thermometer can be a useful tool. I recommend the popular and inexpensive Vicks oral thermometer, and taking oral or rectal readings (pick one or the other, don't go back and forth between the two!). It's good to get a reading first thing in the day to see where you're at. You should see the temperature rise after meals and peak in the late afternoon and early evening – hopefully at a temperature between 98.6 and 99.6. That may seem like a longshot as you are starting out, but keep with it. Very few people fail to respond to my general information without seeing a noticeable rise in body temperature.

Another tool that I do not recommend unless you need it, but may be very handy if you are running into trouble, is a refractometer. A refractometer is a simple tool. You just put a single drop or two of urine on the panel, hold the refractometer up to a light source, and check the reading. Staying out of the overly-diluted zone below about 2.0 brix is life-changing for many people with a history of having many clear urinations daily. I find that simply seeing the connection that often exists between crazy mood states or lifelong illnesses and a reading on a refractometer is enough to transform a person's outlook on his or her illness, and realize that there is really something physiologically going on. That it's not just "in your head."

For less than $30 you can find an acceptable refractometer. The best are the ones with a 0-10% scale as opposed to the more common 0-32% scale. But either will do. Track your daily fluctuations and learn what it feels like when you are "crashing" and it won't be long before you discover your own ideal "zone." Not much more to it.

References

"A Solution to Reducing Inflammation"
http://scienceblog.com/56744/

Rehydran-N Details
http://drugbase.org/drugs/drug_details.php?drugid=1722

"Sodium Intakes Around the World"
http://www.who.int/dietphysicalactivity/Elliot-brown-2007.pdf

"Hyponatremia associated with large-bone fracture in elderly patients"
http://www.springerlink.com/content/g1x5416r83581632/?MUD=MP

"Ingestive Behavior: Drinking"
http://home.epix.net/~tcannon1/Physioweek5.htm

"Intravenous versus Oral Rehydration: Which is best for your athletes?"
http://www.mshsl.org/mshsl/students/rehydration.htm

"Isotonic, hypertonic, hypotonic or water: which sports drink is best for soccer players?"
http://www.footy4kids.co.uk/sports_drink.htm

"Twenty-Four-Hour Urinary Sodium Excretion and Postural Orthostatic Tachycardia Syndrome"
http://www.jpeds.com/article/S0022-3476(12)00112-6/abstract

"Sodium Intake Among Adults – United States 2005-2006"

http://www.cdc.gov/mmwr/preview/mmwrhtml/mm5924a4.htm

"Restoring Blood Volume"
http://www.ncbi.nlm.nih.gov/pmc/articles/PMC1701158/pdf/brm
edj02298-0064a.pdf

"The mysterious origins of the '8 glasses of water a day' rule"
http://www.mindthesciencegap.org/2012/10/22/you-need-to-
drink-8-glasses-of-water-a-day-a-history-lesson/

"Thyroid Disease and the Heart"
http://circ.ahajournals.org/content/116/15/1725.full

"Low urinary sodium is associated with greater risk of myocardial
infarction among treated hypertensive men"
http://www.ncbi.nlm.nih.gov/pubmed?term=%22Hypertension%22
%5BJour%5D+AND+1995%5Bpdat%5D+AND+urinary+sodium
&TransSchema=title&cmd=detailssearch

"Fatal and Nonfatal Outcomes, Incidence of Hypertension, and
Blood Pressure Changes in Relation to Urinary Sodium Excretion"
http://jama.jamanetwork.com/article.aspx?articleid=899663

"Water: swelling, tension, pain, fatigue, aging"
http://raypeat.com/articles/articles/water.shtml

"Salt, Energy, Metabolic Rate, and Longevity"
http://raypeat.com/articles/articles/salt.shtml

"TSH, temperature, pulse rate, and other indicators in
hypothyroidism"
http://raypeat.com/articles/articles/hypothyroidism.shtml

"Coconut Oil"
http://raypeat.com/articles/articles/coconut-oil.shtml

"Water Intoxication"
http://en.wikipedia.org/wiki/Water_intoxication

"It's Time to End the War on Salt"
http://www.scientificamerican.com/article.cfm?id=its-time-to-end-the-war-on-salt

"Urine Specific Gravity"
http://books.google.com/books?id=KMcIPJeqgC8C&pg=PA34&lpg=PA34&dq=1.012+refractometer+urine&source=bl&ots=WOHd12Rfjk&sig=2oGe3M0QkNhUy1TexPgDmOgKLAY&hl=en&sa=X&ei=AcQqT_zAJ4q3twfBh-DlDw&ved=0CJEBEOgBMAU#v=onepage&q=1.012%20refractometer%20urine&f=false

"NSG Precision Cells Releases Revolutionary Digital Specific Gravity Urine Refractometers"
http://www.prweb.com/releases/2011/6/prweb8569085.htm

"Specific Gravity to Brix Conversion Table"
http://www.winning-homebrew.com/specific-gravity-to-brix.html

"Hyponatremia"
http://en.wikipedia.org/wiki/Hyponatremia

"Hyponatremic Seizure Following ECT"
http://www.breggin.com/ECT/HypntrmcSzrFllwgECTcasereport.pdf

"Hyponatremia and Seizures presenting in the first two years of life"
http://www.ncbi.nlm.nih.gov/pubmed/3842164?dopt=Abstract

"Hyponatremic Seizures Secondary to Oral Water Intoxication in Infancy: Association With Commercial Bottled Drinking Water"
http://pediatrics.aappublications.org/content/100/6/e4.full

"Management of hyponatremic seizures in children with hypertonic saline: a safe and effective strategy"
http://www.ncbi.nlm.nih.gov/pubmed/2055051

"Oral Water Intoxication in Infants. An American Epidemic."
http://www.ncbi.nlm.nih.gov/pubmed/1877579?dopt=Abstract

"Seizures and Hypothermia due to dietary water intoxication in infants"
http://www.ncbi.nlm.nih.gov/pubmed/3563573?dopt=Abstract

"Association between obesity and reduced body temperature in dogs"
http://www.nature.com/ijo/journal/v35/n8/full/ijo2010253a.html

"Man (26) died after months on low-salt diet"
http://www.herald.ie/news/courts/man-26-died-after-months-on-lowsalt-diet-3228358.html

About the Author

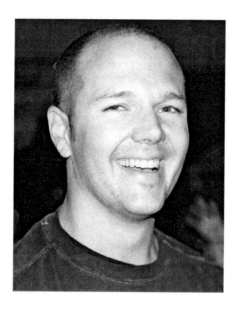

Matt Stone is the founder of 180DegreeHealth. He is an independent health researcher and bestselling author of more than 15 books, including *Eat for Heat*, a #1 Amazon bestselling book since its debut in December, 2012. Most of his research has drawn him towards metabolic rate and how many basic functions (digestion, reproduction, aging, immunity, inflammation, mood, circulation, sleep) perform better when metabolic rate is optimized. He is most notable for his criticisms of extreme diets and exposing many false diet industry claims, as well as his works on raising metabolic rate through simple changes in diet and lifestyle. You can keep up with Matt's at http://www.180degreehealth.com and reading his many books available only at Amazon.

CPSIA information can be obtained at www.ICGtesting.com
Printed in the USA
BVOW04s2111021214

377615BV00007B/430/P